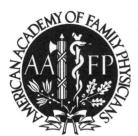

THE ACADEMY COLLECTION
Quick Reference Guides for Family Physicians

D1236078

Management of Adult Urgencies and Emergencies

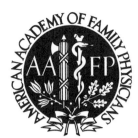

THE ACADEMY COLLECTION
Quick Reference Guides for Family Physicians

Management of Adult Urgencies and Emergencies

RICHARD B. BIRRER, M.D., M.P.H., F.A.A.F.P., F.A.C.E.P.

Professor of Clinical Family Medicine
Department of Family Medicine
State University of New York Health Science Center
Brooklyn, New York;
Chief Medical Officer and Senior Vice President
St. Joseph's Regional Medical Center
Paterson, New Jersey

Series Medical Editor
RICHARD SADOVSKY, M.D., M.S.

Associate Professor of Family Medicine
State University of New York Health Science Center
Brooklyn, New York

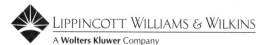

LIPPINCOTT WILLIAMS & WILKINS
A **Wolters Kluwer** Company

Philadelphia · Baltimore · New York · London
Buenos Aires · Hong Kong · Sydney · Tokyo

Acquisitions Editor: Richard Winters
Developmental Editor: Jenny Kim
Production Editor: Christiana Sahl
AAFP Project Manager: Leigh McKinney
Manufacturing Manager: Benjamin Rivera
Cover Designer: Mark Lerner
Compositor: Lippincott Williams & Wilkins Desktop Division
Printer: R.R.Donnelley–Crawfordsville

© 2001 by LIPPINCOTT WILLIAMS & WILKINS
530 Walnut Street
Philadelphia, PA 19106 USA
LWW.com

Printed in the USA

Library of Congress Cataloging-in-Publication Data

Management of adult urgencies and emergencies / [edited by] Richard B. Birrer.
    p. ; cm.—(The academy collection—quick reference guides for family physicians)
    Includes bibliographical references and index.
    ISBN 0-7817-2055-9
    1. Medical emergencies—Handbooks, manuals, etc. 2. Family medicine—Handbooks, manuals, etc. I. Birrer, Richard B. II. Series.

RC86.8 .O35 2001
616.02′5—dc21

                          2001029059

10 9 8 7 6 5 4 3 2 1

CONTENTS

CONTRIBUTING AUTHORS

Fitzgerald Alcindor, M.D.
Attending Physician, Emergency Medicine
Northshore University Hospital
Manhasset, New York

Richard B. Birrer, M.D., M.P.H., F.A.A.F.P., F.A.C.E.P.
Professor of Clinical Family Medicine
Department of Family Medicine
State University of New York Health Science Center
Brooklyn, New York;
Chief Medical Officer and Senior Vice President
St. Joseph's Regional Medical Center
Paterson, New Jersey

Lloyd A. Darlow, M.D., F.A.A.F.P.
Clinical Assistant Professor, Department of Family Practice
University of Rochester School of Medicine and Dentistry
Rochester, New York;
Attending Physician, Departments of Family Practice
  and Emergency Medicine
Cayuga Medical Center
Ithaca, New York

Shaikh Hasan, M.D., F.A.A.F.P.
Assistant Professor of Family Medicine
Cornell University School of Medicine
New York, New York;
Attending Physician, Emergency Medicine
Brooklyn Hospital
Brooklyn, New York

James E. Nahlik, M.D.
Associate Clinical Professor, Department of Community and
  Family Medicine
Saint Louis University School of Medicine
St. Louis, Missouri;
Chief, Department of Family Practice
Missouri Baptist Medical Center
St. Louis, Missouri

Paul R. Pfeiffer, D.O.
Lafayette Grand Hospital
St. Louis, Missouri

Vicken Y. Totten, M.D., M.S., F.A.C.E.P., F.A.A.F.P.
Director of Research Attending, Emergency Medicine
Catholic Medical Centers of Brooklyn and Queens, Inc.
Jamaica, New York

Michael Tretola, E.M.T-P., M.P.A.
Administrator, Outpatient Services
St. Vincent's Catholic Medical Centers
Queens, New York

ACKNOWLEDGMENTS

··

I am very grateful to the staffs of the American Academy of Family Physicians (Richard Sadovsky, M.D., Susanna Guzman, and Leigh McKinney) and Lippincott Williams & Wilkins (Richard Winters, Alexandra Anderson, Jenny Kim, and Christiana Sahl) for their assistance and support throughout the preparation of this book.

A special thanks goes to my author colleagues, whose commitment and energy made this effort worthwhile.

PREFACE

· ·

With the continued evolution and solidification of the family practice specialty, interest in the management of office urgencies and emergencies has grown. For the last several years, the topic has attracted 'sell-out' crowds at the AAFP Annual Scientific Assembly. Family physicians, whether located in the rural, suburban, or urban parts of our country, have always handled such problems as part of the comprehensive nature of the specialty. Now, with the emergence of the basic and clinical science of emergency medicine, family physicians want and need to know how to evaluate and treat an urgently or emergently ill patient who presents in the office setting. The purpose of this book is to provide the busy family physician with a practical guide to a fundamental, evidence-based approach for office medical crises.

Richard B. Birrer

SERIES INTRODUCTION

Family practice is a unique clinical specialty encompassing a philosophy of care rather than a modality of care provided to a specific segment of the population. This philosophy of providing longitudinal care for persons of all ages in the complete context of their physical, emotional, and social environments was modeled by general practitioners, the parents of our modern specialty. To provide this kind of care, the family physician needs a broad knowledge base, appropriate evaluation tools, effective interventions, and patient education.

The knowledge base needed by a family physician is extraordinarily large. The American Academy of Family Physicians and other organizations provide clinical education to practitioners through conferences and journals. Individual family physicians have written journal articles about specific clinical topics or have tried to cover the broad knowledge base of family medicine in a single volume. The former are helpful, but may cover only a narrow segment of medicine, while the latter may not provide the depth needed to be useful in actual patient care.

The Academy Collection: Quick Reference Guides for Family Physicians is a series of books designed to assist family physicians with the broad knowledge base unique to our specialty. The books in this series have all been written by practicing family physicians who have special interest in the topics, and the chapters have been formatted to provide easy access to information needed at varying stages in the physician-patient encounter. Each volume is unique because each author has personalized the volume and provided a unique family physician perspective.

This series is not meant to be a final reference for the family physician who seeks a comprehensive text. The series also does not cover every topic that may be encountered by the family physician. The series does offer, in a depth deemed appropriate by the authors, the information needed by the physician to handle the majority of patient encounters. The series also provides information to make patient care a combined doctor-patient effort. Specific patient education materials have been included where appropriate. Readers can contact the American Academy of Family Physicians Foundation for other resources.

The topics selected for *The Academy Collection* were chosen based on what family physicians said they needed. The books cover office procedures, conditions of aging, challenging diagnoses, musculoskeletal problems, occupational medicine, children's health, gastrointestinal problems, and women's health issues.

I welcome your comments. Please contact me at the American Academy of Family Physicians with your suggestions (Rick Sadovsky, MD, Series Editor, *The Academy Collection*, c/o AAFP, 11400 Tomahawk Creek Parkway, Leawood, KS 66211-2672; e-mail: academycollection@aafp.org). This collection is meant to be useful to you and your patients.

Richard Sadovsky, M.D., M.S.
Series Editor

CHAPTER 1

Management of Adult Urgencies and Emergencies

An Overview

Richard B. Birrer

The heart of family practice is providing continuous, coordinated care. In this role family physicians are sometimes requested to attend to medical or surgical urgencies and to consider the worrisome possibility of a true office emergency. Given the rarity and complexity of emergencies, being adequately prepared for them can seem a daunting task. Yet this preparation is required of family physicians as part of their broad scope of care.

Data from the National Ambulatory Medical Care Survey indicate that about 55% of office visits are for acute problems and that 2% of these visits require hospital admission—an incidence rate of about 1% per year. Approximately 75% of all acute visits are routine or nonurgent, 24%-25% are urgent; and less than 1% are emergent. The average office practice experiences one to two emergencies per month. Trauma diagnoses involving the skin, eye, and musculoskeletal system account for 60% of emergencies. Medical urgencies, such as chest and abdominal pain, headache, respiratory distress, dizziness, syncope, dehydration, and hypertension or hypotension, account for the remaining 40%. Cardiopulmonary arrest occurs in 1 of 15,000-20,000 patient visits or in 0.7-1.2% of all true emergencies. In a busy solo practice, this translates to one arrest every 3-4 years. Similarly, practices providing the full spectrum of women's health care will see obstetric emergencies, such as preeclampsia, ectopic pregnancy, and third-trimester bleeding. Physicians who provide care for many children will also see a number of office emergencies. Certain byproducts of managed care—an increased frequency of outpatient procedures and in the use of conscious sedation, primary care physicians acting as gatekeepers, and increased ambulatory management of complex medical problems—are probably going to increase the likelihood of the office presentation of urgencies and emergencies. Also, aging of the general population is likely to cause the number of office emergencies to rise.

Surveys have indicated that specialists in pediatrics and dentistry are more likely to diagnose and treat office emergencies (1–7). As many as 62% of office-based pediatricians reported at least one urgency (treatment required within several hours) per week (8). The incidence of life-threatening emergencies is approximately 1 per physician-year (9). The annual incidence of non-life–threatening emergencies (e.g., angina or a long-bone fracture) is about 20 times higher. A study of 114 pediatricians found that the annual risk of a patient with a severe life-threatening emergency presenting to the office setting ranged from 1 to 250 (to 23 visits per month). The frequency by emergency diagnoses was 0–2 cardiac arrests, 0–8 endocrine, 0–11 status epilepticus, 0–50 shock, 0–500 upper airway obstruction, 1–75 status asthmaticus, and 0–250 for trauma (10). Very busy practices can experience more than 100 emergencies annually. These catastrophes frequently present to the office during the late afternoon and early evening.

Studies have documented that most practices are inadequately prepared for emergencies and lack crucial equipment or appropriate life support training (8–12). Crucial supplies, such as oxygen, intravenous catheters and fluids, bag–valve-mask, nebulizers, and epinephrine, are not available 30%–40% of the time. Staff members in about 70% of office practices have minimal training for status asthmaticus management; only one-third are prepared for other emergencies. Almost no office practice is prepared for a cardiac arrest. The most common reasons for lack of readiness, in order of frequency, are that (a) emergencies are rare, (b) the practice is busy, (c) the hospital is nearby, (d) the staff is inadequately equipped and trained, and (e) the cost of preparedness is too high. Ironically, up to 90% of these emergencies could be managed and resolved in the office setting at an annual cost savings of several hundred dollars (10,13). The likelihood that family physicians, particularly those in rural areas and/or those with a busy pediatrics or obstetrics component, will see an office emergency or urgency is very real. For this reason alone, having the office staff receive the appropriate training and keeping the necessary equipment on hand are essential. Available evidence suggests that early and aggressive intervention in these cases can have a profound impact on outcome and survival.

The intent of this reference guide is to provide the busy office-based physician with a practical compendium for diagnosing and treating common urgencies and emergencies in primary care. Critical diagnostic criteria, treatment principles, and referral guidelines are provided as a template for efficient evaluation and decision making in a time-pressured situation. The outline format of the guide provides easy access to sections covering chief complaint, clinical manifestations, risk factors, epidemiologic factors, pathophysiologic factors, diagnosis, referral, management, follow-up/prognosis, and patient education/prevention. Ample illustrations and figures are used for medications, differential diagnoses, decision algorithms, procedures, and pathology. Suggested readings and appendices are also provided for further clarification. The authors are board-certified in family medicine and emergency medicine, and they practice and teach both specialties.

REFERENCES

1. The emergency physician and the office-based pediatrician: an EMSC team. American Academy of Pediatrics. Committee on Pediatric Emergency Medicine. *Pediatrics* 1998;101:936-937.

2. Buyre MT, Gobetti JP, Plezia R. A basic approach to management of medical emergencies in the dental office. Part 1. *J Mich Dent Assoc* 1998;80: 34-43.

3. Buyre MT, Gobetti JP, Plezia R. Medical emergencies in the dental office. Part 2. *J Mich Dent Assoc* 1998;80:52, 56-59.

4. Kaplan BR. Treatment of medical emergencies for the general practitioner. *R I Dent J* 1994;27:5-7.

5. Lipp M, Kubota Y, Malamed SF, et al. Management of an emergency: to be prepared for the unwanted event. *Anesth Pain Control Dent* 1992;1: 90-102.

6. Malamed SF. Back to basics: emergency medicine in dentistry. *J Calif Dent Assoc* 1997;25:285-286, 288-294.

7. Schexnayder SM, Schexnayder RE. 911 in your office: preparations to keep emergencies from becoming catastrophes. *Pediatr Ann* 1996;25: 664-666, 668, 670, passim.

8. Fuchs S, Jaffe DM, Christoffel KK. Pediatric emergencies in office practices: prevalence and office preparedness. *Pediatrics* 1989;83:931-939.

9. Altieri M, Bellet J, Scott H. Preparedness for pediatric emergencies encountered in the practitioner's office. *Pediatrics* 1990;85:710-714.

10. Flores G, Weinstock DJ. The preparedness of pediatricians for emergencies in the office. *Arch Pediatr Adolesc Med* 1996;150:249-256.

11. Schweich PJ, DeAngelis C, Duggan AK. Preparedness of practicing pediatricians to manage emergencies. *Pediatrics* 1991;88:223-229.

12. Shetty AK, Hutchinson SW, Mangat R, Peck GQ. Preparedness of practicing pediatricians in Louisiana to manage emergencies. *South Med J* 1998; 91:745-748.

13. Herranz JB, Hernandez MR, Caceres GR, et al. Pediatric emergencies in a community health center (in Spanish). *An Esp Pediatr* 1997;47:591-594.

CHAPTER 2

The General Approach to Urgencies and Emergencies

Prepare for the Worst, Hope for the Best

Richard B. Birrer and Michael Tretola

As in most things, prevention is surely the best strategy when dealing with office-based medical emergencies. Physicians should anticipate complications, such as drug allergies and hypersensitivities, and should have the right equipment in the right place at the right time (1). Acquiring certification in basic cardiac life support (BCLS), advanced cardiac life support (ACLS), advanced trauma life support (ATLS), and pediatric advanced life support (PALS) is a necessary first step, but failure to practice these skills both individually and as a team leads to skill atrophy (2,3). As a matter of fact, research has shown that medical staff must respond to or practice one code situation per week to maintain performance capacity The literature is very clear that the major problems in most code situations are the failure to do the priority basics (airway stabilization and compressions) and the lack of team coordination. Therefore, training, written plans, periodic drills, and critiques are probably more important than current certification.

The family physician should assess the readiness of his or her office staff for pediatric and adult urgencies and emergencies. An assessment of basic and advanced life support training should be undertaken, and the required levels of certification should be maintained. Drills and protocols for different emergency scenarios (e.g., cardiac arrest, respiratory distress, trauma, shock, etc.) should be established with training, equipment needs, and responsibilities that are clearly defined for professional and nonprofessional staff. The strategy will be more flexible and more effective if all team members are involved in planning. A review system for evaluation and improvement should be established for all emergency responses. A formal network of providers and their liaisons should be identified and should include an emergency department (ED), a hospital, colleagues, and home health care. Lastly, protocols for communication with community response agencies (telephone hot-line numbers for fire, police, ambulance, poison control) should be established in advance and maintained. Given the obvious fact that a misdiagnosed or inappropriately treated urgency or emergency can have devastating clinical and legal consequences, the wisest approach is *semper paratus,* meaning that one should always be prepared. Physicians should be ACLS-certified, and support staff should be current in BCLS. Each practice should have, at the very least, basic office equipment and medications (Appendix 1). In addition, conducting periodic office test runs to maintain proficiency and to maximize emergency response time and behaviors is important. These drills should initially be conducted without patients; subsequent drills can include patients, if feasible. Debriefing and evaluation (e.g., of technique and timeline) after drills and real emergencies are essential.

A general checklist that can help normalize and reinforce actions during drills and actual emergencies is outlined below.

PRIORITIZE

Do the ABCDEs: airway, breathing, circulation, disability, and exposure.

Fundamental lifesaving interventions are mandatory before beginning any detailed evaluation or treatment protocol.

IDENTIFY

Consider the worst case first. Although clinicians are trained to consider the most common possibilities first, the urgency and the unexpected nature of a medical crisis calls for consideration of both the obviously dramatic and the insidiously subtle diagnostic possibility. The most serious possibilities are at the top of the list, and their workup takes precedence. For example, pulmonary embolism should be considered a high priority in a 38-year-old woman who presents with shortness of breath, who smokes, and who is taking an oral contraceptive.

RULE OUT

The approach to the diagnostic and management options must be systematic. A methodical history, physical, and ancillary diagnostic workup must begin with vital signs. Fetal heart tones should be obtained if the patient is at least 12 weeks pregnant. After the primary survey, begin the secondary survey or physical examination, including a history that is AMPLE (allergies, medications, past history, last meal, events leading to the current illness).

BE VIGILANT

Very often, serial examinations (i.e., repeated evaluations) and prolonged observation (i.e., several hours) reveal an elusive diagnosis outside the routine inventory. For instance, shortness of breath in an 83-year-old may be the presenting and only complaint of an evolving myocardial infarction. Good emergency medicine rules out all considerations and does not jump at the most obvious explanation. Major misdiagnoses have occurred because a simpler or a more familiar diagnosis was made. Bear in mind that a patient with a seemingly minor illness can suddenly decompensate, resulting in a major medical catastrophe.

COORDINATE

Decide in advance who is in charge when an emergency occurs. Although this is usually the physician, a physician's assistant or office nurse may be the point person when the physician is out of the office. Cross-training of office staff is an essential element of a disaster plan that maximizes response flexibility.

FOCUS

The true bottom line for clinical care in a high-pressure situation is to treat the patient and not the laboratory, radiograph, or monitor. Repeat any study whose results do not make sense. For example, a child may look and act normal but may actually be on the way to clinical shock.

COMMUNICATE

Let the patient and family members know, in nonmedical terms, what you think and what you are planning to do. Keep your staff and colleagues (consultants and referring physician) informed. Do not minimize the seriousness of the circumstances. Know personal limitations and ask for assistance when necessary.

MAINTAIN EQUANIMITY

Calmness in a crisis situation does more for the patient, family, friends, and staff performance than any other single factor. Deliberate action, an even voice, and a positive attitude set an example that the staff will follow.

DOCUMENT

Keeping a careful and detailed record of the diagnostic and therapeutic events that occur during the emergency is essential. Record the essence of conversations with patient, family, consultants, and managed care representatives. The chart should reflect the logistics of the actions and thinking. Notes, particularly orders, should be timed. In terms of documentation, the bottom line is, "if it isn't written in the medical chart, it wasn't done." Most successful malpractice cases are based on poor documentation.

DISPOSITION

Before discharging the patient to go home, ruling out all underlying critical illnesses is imperative. Ambulance transportation must be arranged for a patient with an emergency or for a patient who requires hospital admission. Although the Consolidated Omnibus Rehabilitation Act—Emergency Medical Transportation Act regulations allow the transport of an unstable patient to a facility where the clinical outcome is likely to be more favorable, every effort must be made to stabilize the patient in the office setting. Do not interrupt lifesaving interventions in favor of private vehicle transportation. Call the ambulance service, copy all records and diagnostic studies (electrocardiograms, radiographs, and the like), contact the receiving institution and discuss the case with the on-call physician, and then send the patient. Remember that the physician is the patient's advocate.

The following is a summary of current life support methodology:

Assess for Responsiveness

What is seen at the emergency scene or office setting? How does the patient appear on first contact? Is he or she alert and oriented or stuporous and obtunded? A brief primary survey assesses responsiveness. Does the patient respond to gentle tapping or shaking? Does the patient respond to the question, "Are you okay?"

Activate EMS

Call 911 if the patient is unresponsive.

Airway

The first priority is always to establish airway patency. A head-tilt chin lift or jaw-thrust maneuver should be performed because tongue occlusion is the most common cause of airway obstruction in the unconscious victim. The jaw-thrust technique is the safest intervention in a patient with potential neck injury. Remove any foreign material (e.g., vomitus) from the mouth. Insert an oropharyngeal airway if a comatose patient demonstrates spontaneous respirations. Intubation in the office setting should only be attempted by a physician who has the appropriate skills and equipment.

FOREIGN BODY MANAGEMENT

Complete airway obstruction in an adult is treated with the Heimlich maneuver, which consists of several quick, forceful upward thrusts applied well below the xyphoid process but above the umbilicus. Women in the third trimester of pregnancy or morbidly obese patients are treated with chest thrusts. For patients who are unconscious or who become so, the following sequence is recommended: (a) perform a finger sweep of the open mouth; (b) attempt to ventilate; (c) perform the Heimlich maneuver up to five times if unable to ventilate; (d) repeat finger sweep; (e) attempt to ventilate; and (f) reperform the sequence of Heimlich maneuver, finger sweep, and ventilation attempt as often as is necessary. Direct visualization of the hypopharynx with a tongue blade and a light or laryngoscope should be attempted early. A Kelly clamp or Magill forceps can be used to remove a visualized foreign body.

Breathing

If spontaneous respirations are not detected, provide ventilation with a bag-valve device; or, if this is unavailable, perform mouth-to-mouth rescue breathing using a barrier device to prevent the spread of infectious disease. In adults, 2 initial breaths followed by 10–12 breaths per minute are appropriate. One hundred percent oxygen should be given as soon as possible.

Circulation

Chest compression at the rate of 80–100 per minute for the average adult is initiated if the patient is pulseless. The sternum is depressed 1–2 inches with each compression. If only one rescuer is present, 15 compressions are followed by 2 breaths. For two-rescuer cardiopulmonary resuscitation (CPR), the compression-to-ventilation ratio is 5:1.

INTRAVENOUS ACCESS

After ensuring airway patency and breathing adequacy and addressing the risk of serious hemorrhage, intravenous (IV) access is a major priority in the management of any emergency. IV access can be used for phlebotomy, for delivery of medication and fluids, and for nutrition (dextrose, etc.). Most commonly, an IV line is established as a precautionary measure in patients who have a potentially life-threatening condition.

EQUIPMENT

The recommended equipment used for performing IV access is shown in Table 2.1. A variety of catheters can be used to establish IV access. However,

T ABLE 2.1. Equipment needed to establish an intravenous access line

- Catheter
- Tape
- Tourniquet
- Gauze sponges
- Alcohol swabs
- Latex gloves
- Saline lock or fluid administration set
- Veniguard or similar device

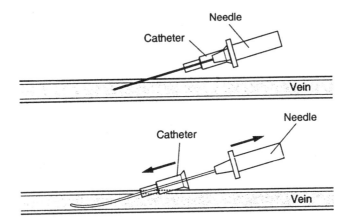

FIGURE 2.1. Inserting the catheter into the vein. Insert the catheter bevel up into the vein at a low angle. Insert the catheter-needle assembly into the vein. Watch for blood to "flash" back into the needle chamber. This indicates that the catheter is in the vein lumen.

the needle most frequently used during emergency care is the "catheter over the needle" device, which is preassembled with a plastic catheter over the metal needle (4). The needle is inserted into the vein and then is withdrawn as the catheter is advanced into the lumen (Fig. 2.1). The needle is removed and is placed in a sharp's container. The IV tubing or saline lock is then connected to the hub of the plastic catheter.

SITE SELECTION

The site at which an IV line is inserted should be determined by a brief examination of the selected area to ensure that the vein is straight with healthy subcutaneous tissue. The dorsal aspect of the hand and the antecubital fos-

T ABLE 2.2. Steps in establishing an intravenous line

- Place tourniquet proximal to the insertion site.
- Heed universal safety precautions (gloves).
- After locating the vein, swab the site with alcohol, making increasingly larger concentric circles.
- Stabilize the vein distal to the insertion site.
- With the needle bevel side up, enter the vein from the side or from above. There should be blood return to the catheter.
- Advance the catheter and remove the needle.
- Remove the tourniquet.
- Attach the infusion set or saline lock.
- Cover the site.
- Secure the IV line with tape.

sae are the most common sites for obtaining access. The steps for IV line insertion are listed in Table 2.2. Once established, the site should be monitored frequently for complications, such as infiltration and/or infection.

Defibrillation

The success of early defibrillation in cardiac arrest has been proved time and again. The American Heart Association (AHA) states that "early defibrillation should be considered in free-standing settings where employees or the public are likely to seek first assistance from healthcare personnel." Furthermore, the AHA now considers defibrillation a BCLS skill. However, owning a manually operated combination monitor-defibrillator is probably cost prohibitive and impractical for most offices. Maintenance and training limitations make this device unattractive for most family practice settings. Constant reviews in rhythm interpretation and use of the machine are necessary for proper operation. Additionally, U.S. Food and Drug Administration (FDA) regulations require annual inspection of such devices by a biomedical service. Use of the manually operated defibrillator in the practice setting is usually limited by statute to the physician, registered nurse, or physician's assistant. However, technological advances during the past decade have produced an innovative device called the automated external defibrillator (AED). This machine eliminates the need for user interpretation of cardiac dysrhythmias. Voice prompts guide the user through a preset protocol. In many cases, the use of lithium batteries allows the machine to remain unused, yet fully charged, for 5–7 years. AEDs are a relatively inexpensive and effective alternative for physicians who want access to a defibrillator. Currently, several brands are available, with prices ranging from $2,000 to $5,000. In most states, nonprofessional staff are permitted to use this device under the guidance of a physician and after completion of a 3- to 4-hour training program. Recently, the AHA developed a simple curriculum, called Heartsaver/AED, to teach laypersons CPR and the AED technique.

Disability

Perform a secondary survey, particularly noting neurologic status.

Expose

In a possible trauma situation, removal of all of the patient's clothing is an absolute must because total inspection of the patient's body is required for thorough assessment. For example, a small stab or bullet wound in the lower back or buttock would be the likely cause of unexplained shock.

MEDICATIONS

The well-prepared office has a number of emergency medications available in a secure but easily accessible place. The most commonly stocked medications, along with their uses and dosages, are listed in Table 2.3.

T ABLE 2.3.   Common medications used for resuscitation and other emergencies

Medication	Use	Common adult dosage
Oxygen	Correct potential or symptomatic hypoxia	Nasal cannula 2–6 L/min Mask 8–15 L/min BVM or pocket mask 15 L/min
Epinephrine (Sus-Phrine, EpiPen)	Cardiac arrest	1.0 mg of a 1:10,000 solution every 3–5 min, IV bolus. If still no change in rhythm, increase to 3.0 mg every 3–5 min
	Anaphylactic reaction	0.01 mg/kg of a 1:1,000 solution
Nitroglycerine (Nitrostat, NitroQuick)	Ischemic chest pain; congestive heart failure	0.3, 0.4, or 0.5 mg, sublingually. Dosage may be repeated at 5 min intervals up to a total of three tablets
Furosemide (Lasix)	Congestive heart failure	0.5–1.0 mg/kg IV bolus initially; 2.0 mg/kg in total
Dextrose	Hypoglycemia; unconscious patient; unknown cause	25 g, IV bolus
Metaproterenol 5% (Alupent)	Asthma, COPD	Via nebulizer over 5–10 min
Methylprednisolone (Solu-Medrol, A-Methapred)	Asthma, COPD	10–40 mg over one to several minutes
Proparacaine HCL 0.5% (Alcaine, Opthaine, Ophthetic)	Chemical eye injuries	1 drop every 5–10 min for a total of 5–7 drops
Aspirin	Myocardial infarction	160–325 mg PO
Naloxone (Narcan)	Reversal of narcotic depression	0.4–2 mg IV bolus; may repeat at 2–3 minute intervals
Oxytocin (Pitocin, Syntocinon)[a]	Control postpartum uterine bleeding	10–40 units (0.5–1.0 mL) added to 1,000 mL of nonhydrating diluent; maximum dosage of 40 units

BVM, bag-valve-mask; COPD, chronic obstructive pulmonary disease.
[a]If actively practicing obstetrics.

Pediatric Medication Dosages

The importance of using a commercially prepared reference chart for determining pediatric dosages in the case of an emergency cannot be overemphasized. A high level of anxiety often accompanies emergency cases that involve a pediatric patient. Advance preparation helps to avoid medication errors as physicians struggle in a crisis to calculate weight-related dosing. Several manufacturers produce a reference chart of pediatric values at a reasonable cost (under $20).

Costs of Updating Medications

A periodic review of medication expiration dates (usually every 2 years) should be performed by one of the staff members, and replacements should be secured. The physician can expect to spend about $50 per year to maintain the medication stock.

GRIEF MANAGEMENT

Despite the best efforts and well-directed intentions, a patient's life may be lost; or his or her quality of life may be adversely affected (major trauma with limb loss, spontaneous abortion, rape, and so forth). A prepared physician has usually come to grips with his or her own mortality, recognizes vulnerability and associated feelings, and understands the normal grieving process. The physician should take the lead role in facilitating the grief reactions of the patient and staff members by first identifying and reconciling feelings of inadequacy and guilt about the outcome. Early, culturally sensitive communication with the patient and family members is critical. By recognizing feelings of anger and guilt in all those who are involved, the physician allows the grieving process to take place. The physician can decrease feelings of guilt through reassurance that the outcome was most likely unavoidable (e.g., in cases of sudden infant death syndrome).

REFERENCES

1. Klinzig G, McClure C. Could your office cope with a disaster? *Fam Pract Manage* 1999;6(8): 26–30.
2. Chandra NC, Hazinski MF, eds. *Basic life support for healthcare providers*. Dallas: American Heart Association, 1997.
3. Cummins RO, ed. *Advanced cardiac life support*. Dallas: American Heart Association, 1998.
4. Roberts PW. *Useful procedures in medical practice*. Philadelphia: Lea and Febiger, 1986.

CHAPTER 3

Pulmonary

Vicken Y. Totten

Only a few pulmonary disorders can quickly become life threatening in the office. Each disorder manifests with difficulty breathing, or *dyspnea*. (Dyspnea is abnormal respiration that is experienced as unpleasant and is concomitant with excessive respiratory labor.) A few simple tools will help distinguish among these disorders: a stethoscope, a pulse oximeter, a peak flowmeter, and a chest radiograph, in addition to an appropriate index of suspicion. Some disorders can be managed completely in the office; for others, treatment may be initiated in the office while emergency medical services are on the way. This chapter will cover the initial office treatment of persons with selected pulmonary emergencies: severe asthma, pneumothorax, acute pulmonary edema, and pulmonary embolism.

SEVERE ASTHMA

By definition asthma is a disease of *recurrent* bronchospasm. However, it is also a chronic, immune-mediated disease characterized by airway hyper-responsiveness that causes reversible obstruction and by airway inflammation that is manifested by secretion and edema.

The office diagnosis can be either straightforward or remarkably obscure. Asthma should be suspected when the patient complains of chronic or seasonal cough, nocturnal cough, or posttussive vomiting. Some patients complain of chest tightness or dyspnea with a minimal bronchospasm; others insist they feel fine even when objective tests demonstrate profound obstruction (1). Pulmonary function studies with provocation and amelioration remain the gold standard. However, in the office setting, simple peak flow monitoring or even a therapeutic trial of bronchodilators may suggest the diagnosis.

Chief Complaint

A 32-year-old woman presents to the office with a 3-week history of gradually increasing dyspnea, dry cough, and mild respirophasic chest pain. She complains of general chest tightness and dyspnea. She has a 10-pack-year history of smoking and a family history of asthma. She says she outgrew her childhood asthma, which her pediatrician used to treat with "shots."

Clinical Manifestations

The woman seems comfortable at rest, although she talks in short sentences. Occasionally, she has coughing fits, some of which cause her to gag before they terminate.

Physical examination: The patient is afebrile, with a respiratory rate of 18–20/min and a heart rate of 90 beats per minute (bpm). She shows no cyanosis or pallor. On auscultation a few scattered wheezes with globally diminished breath sounds are heard. No pedal edema is found. Pulse oximetry is 94%. Peak expiratory flow rate (PEFR) is 150. You explain to her how to use a metered-dose inhaler (MDI) device and also how much more effective it is with a spacer. After six puffs from an albuterol MDI attached to a spacer, her peak flow is 250.

Epidemiologic Factors

The incidence of asthma is increasing globally, especially in the New York area. Prevalence is increasing in all age groups. The under-20 age group shows the greatest increase (2,3). The reasons for the global increase are not known, but suspected culprits vary widely, including problems ranging from air pollution to cockroach dander and from dust mite feces to lack of intestinal parasites.

Risk Factors

- Atopy
- Family history
- Urban environment
- History of "allergies"
- Bottle-fed rather than breast-fed
- Secondhand smoke exposure
- Crowded living conditions
- Low socioeconomic status

Pathophysiology

Asthma is a state of increased responsiveness of the respiratory tree to irritants. These irritants may be exogenous (e.g., pollen, noxious fumes) or intrinsic (e.g., overactive inflammatory cells, autoimmune immunoglobulins). As the bronchi and bronchioles respond, their smooth muscles contract, narrowing the airway diameter. At almost the same time, leukotrienes signal mast cell degranulation and initiate an inflammatory cascade in the respiratory epithelium. Secretions increase, becoming thicker and more tenacious. This inflammation involves the terminal bronchioles and even the alveoli. As the mucosa thickens from inflammation, the distance between gas and blood in the alveoli increases. Respiratory effort and rate increase to compensate. As air flow increases, secretions inspissate, blocking the smallest airways.

Cough is a prominent symptom that in and of itself predisposes to increasing airway hypersensitivity. Cough is triggered when respiratory cilia are bent either by secretions or simply by contact with the opposite wall of the now-narrowed airway. Air travels in excess of 150 km per second during a cough; coughing can denude patches of respiratory epithelium. As the basement membranes are uncovered, they are exposed to particles that may stimulate a future antigenic or irritative response.

The initial, bronchospastic stage of asthma is easily reversed by bronchodilators; but the next stage, characterized by a fixed narrowing of the airways, does not respond to them. The cascade of inflammation may continue even as the patient feels better after treatment with a beta agonist. By the time the inspissated mucus and cellular debris have caused bronchiolar plugging, the airway obstruction is very difficult to relieve; and death may ensue.

Differential Diagnosis

In children:

- Tracheomalacia
- Aspirated foreign body
- Bronchopulmonary dysplasia
- Croup
- Cystic fibrosis
- Upper respiratory infection
- Unilateral hyperlucent lung syndrome (Swyer–James)
- Bronchitis
- Pneumonia

    In adults:

- Congestive heart failure (CHF)
- Impending acute pulmonary edema (APE)
- Emphysema
- Chronic obstructive pulmonary disease (COPD)
- Foreign body aspiration
- Bronchial neoplasms
- Fungal, viral, or bacterial infection of the airways

Diagnostic Tests

PEFR measurement is generally considered reliable after the age of 5 years, and target PEFR is estimated by patient height. PEFR measurement is simple, noninvasive, and able to be performed at home. Patients should be instructed to measure the PEFR frequently, to know their personal best, and to commence treatment if they note a 20% decrease in PEFR.

Pulse oximetry is easier to perform than PEFR because it requires no patient cooperation. Pulse oximetry is useful for diagnosis but is less useful for making decisions about the need for hospitalization in a child younger than 3 years of age (4). Although usually unnecessary, arterial blood gas (ABG) measurement may be useful in the presence of potentially life-threatening asthma but is seldom available in the office setting.

Chest x-ray also is seldom helpful, except to suggest an alternative diagnosis that may have been misdiagnosed as asthma (such as heart failure, anomalous great vessels, or unilateral pulmonary atresia). The chest x-ray in asthma may show hyperinflation but, in general, should only be obtained when a complication, such as pneumonia or pneumothorax, is suspected.

Referral

The initial and general management of controllable asthma is completely appropriate for the office practitioner: physician, physician's assistant, or nurse practitioner. The patients who should be evaluated by a pulmonologist include those with continuous or recurrent asthma, those who have asthma unresponsive to the three-step treatment (see below), those who have asthma in association with other severe systemic illnesses, or those who suffer a life-threatening pulmonary event. Some patients react to environmental stimulants, such as animal or insect dander, pollens, or certain foods. An allergist may assist in identifying asthma triggers.

Management

Beta agonists have been said to treat the symptoms but steroids, the disease. Fortunately, the modern repertoire of asthma medications has increased to include medications that can prevent or abort the airway reactivity as well: cromones (cromolyn sodium, nedocromil sodium) and leukotriene inhibitors (montelukast [Singulair], zafirlukast [Accolate], zileutron [Zyflo]).

The office treatment of asthma is generally managed in three steps according to the severity of the disease: mild, moderate, or severe. The first step, inhaling beta agonists as needed, is appropriate for patients who have less than one attack per month. The second step, prophylaxis with inhaled steroids or inhaled cromones, is appropriate for persons who have attacks about once a week if untreated. Consider adding ipratropium bromide if the patient may have an element of emphysema. In the third step, inhaled prophylactic medications are combined with oral leukotriene inhibitors. At all stages, an acute exacerbation may be managed with a brief burst of oral steroids. Parenteral steroids have no proven advantage, and no need to taper exists if the therapy lasts less than 14 days. This chapter focuses on the initial management of a severe attack of dyspnea in a patient with known or suspected asthma.

For any patient presenting with acute dyspnea, the first step is evaluating the potential for threat to life. Obtain a PEFR and pulse oximetry reading. A

peak flow of 50% or less than the patient's personal best or a pulse oximeter reading at or below 90% suggests a potential threat to life. The patients
at greatest risk are those who have put off treatment for days to weeks,
patients with severe asthma (defined as daily attacks if untreated), and
patients who have previously been intubated or who are already steroid
dependent. Asthma of abrupt onset is usually more quickly reversed than is
airway obstruction, which develops gradually (see "Pathophysiology"
above).

Modern beta agonists are fairly specific and have less alpha (cardiac)
effect than older drugs (e.g., epinephrine or isoetharine); therefore, they are
considered the first-line treatment in an episode of bronchospasm. Beta agonists are considered safe in pregnancy or even in the presence of severe
heart disease. Tachycardia is usually caused by hypoxemia, not by underlying
cardiac disease or the cardiostimulant effects of beta agonists, and is not a
contraindication to their use.

Over the first hour, administer three unit doses of an inhaled short-acting
beta agonist, such as albuterol, by nebulization or 18 activations from an MDI
attached to a spacer device. Repeat PEFR and pulse oximetry.

Studies have not demonstrated the superiority of nebulization over delivery by an MDI in adults or in children older than 5 years of age unless they
are extremely uncooperative. However, for best effect, an MDI should be
used with a spacer. A number of commercial spacer devices, such as the
AeroChamber, are available; in a pinch, even a foam cup with a hole punched
in the bottom will work. The spacer holds the MDI further from the mouth,
providing an extra few microseconds for the carrier fluid to evaporate,
which decreases the size of the inhaled particles and deposits the drug more
deeply in the respiratory tract. The spacer also diminishes the side-stream
loss of drug. Spacers are recommended for home use because achieving correct coordination and positioning for efficient MDI use can be difficult.
Approximately six activations of an albuterol MDI are equivalent to one unit
dose of nebulized albuterol.

Alternatives to the use of inhaled beta agonists do exist, although these
alternatives are no longer considered first-line therapy. Epinephrine can be
given subcutaneously in a 1:1,000 dilution. Administer 0.3 mL to an adult
(0.01 mg/kg to a child). Epinephrine can also be nebulized in a 1:10,000
solution. Another candidate for nebulization is furosemide (Lasix). Studies
have shown that it is a moderately effective bronchodilator in and of itself; it
also potentiates beta agonistic effects. Ipratropium bromide (Atrovent) is a
quaternary ammonium salt of atropine. It is more effective in chronic
obstructive pulmonary disease (COPD) than in pure bronchospastic asthma,
but it is virtually free of side effects and can be added to each unit dose of
atropine or by MDI, with one puff for every three to six metaproterenol (Alu-
pent) activations. Theophylline has no place in the initial treatment of acute
bronchospasm and has fallen into disfavor for long-term management
because of its side effects and narrow therapeutic window.

Steroids have, in the last 20 years, moved from a position of "drug of last resort" to a firm position in the initial treatment of severe asthma and to part of the regimen of long-term treatment. If the patient has not returned completely to baseline after the first round of beta agonist therapy, steroids can be administered. Beta agonists have no effect on the airway wall inflammation and mucosal edema and have minimal effects on airway debris. Steroids reverse the cascade of inflammation and thus decrease future sensitivity.

The literature does not demonstrate a superiority of parenteral steroids over orally administered systemic steroids, nor does the literature or physiology support any need for a taper if the total duration of steroid administration is less than 14 days. For long-term use or for prevention, inhalation is unequivocally the route of choice.

The appropriate dose of steroids during an acute exacerbation remains more a matter of tradition than of research, but common initial intravenous (IV) doses range from 40 mg to 120 mg of methylprednisolone (Solu-Medrol, A-Methapred); initial oral doses, from 40 mg of prednisone (Meticorten, Deltasone) to 120 mg of methylprednisolone.

After the initial, potentially life-threatening event has been ameliorated, the purpose of asthma treatment is to prevent future attacks. The patient should be told to carry a beta agonist for treatment of acute sudden exacerbations and should also be given instruction in how to prevent attacks. Most prevention medications are inhalants; however, the new antileukotrienes are taken orally, which increases their acceptance. Among inhaled medications are cromones, such as nedocromil (Tilade) or cromolyn (Intal). Cromolyn should be puffed once or twice, four times a day, whereas two puffs of nedocromil can be given on a twice-daily basis. Ipratropium bromide functions as both treatment and prevention. Innumerable inhaled steroids currently are available. Theophylline in its various preparations is now considered a third-line medication, as are oral steroids. Advise the patient about drug–drug interactions with theophylline, especially with erythromycins and antihistamines.

Future directions for asthma treatment or prevention may include the newer antihistamines or other immunomodulatory drugs, as well as environmental control.

Medications for the initial treatment of severe asthma are as follows:

- Beta agonists—treat the symptoms. Begin with three activations of an albuterol or proventil MDI six times (or three unit doses of nebulized albuterol) in 1 hour or less.
- Steroids—treat the disease. Begin with 40–100 mg of methylprednisolone orally; may be repeated in 6 hours and daily thereafter.
- Cromones—stabilize mast cells against degranulation. Have no place in acute management.
- Leukotriene inhibitors—stop one portion of the cascade of inflammation; probably not effective in the first 24 hours of treatment.
- Anticholinergics—suppress excess mucus production; ipatropium bromide by nebulizer can be used acutely.

The acute attack may provide a good teachable moment to initiate discussion of modalities such as environmental manipulation and smoking cessation. Breathing exercises and pursed-lip breathing are no longer considered appropriate, but visualization and hypnosis may still have a place in the management of chronic asthma.

Follow-up

Potential complications of life-threatening asthma include emphysema, pneumothorax or pneumonia, steroid dependency (with its accompanying consequences), and an ever-increasing reactivity to environmental stimulants. Asthmatics are not only more prone to asthma attacks with other illnesses; but, because of the damage to respiratory mucosa, they also are more prone to respiratory infections. In the older asthmatic or patient with COPD, consider that the stress of the attack could precipitate myocardial ischemia or myocardial infarction (MI).

The initial treatment with beta agonists can improve respirations enough to fool both the physician and the patient into thinking that the patient is well before the underlying inflammation has actually subsided. Steroid bursts have a place in the treatment of any significant exacerbation.

Follow-up is essential. Asthma is a life-long disease that can have long periods of quiescence. Home monitoring should primarily consist of peak flow measurement. Many patients are given undated prescriptions for steroids and are instructed by their primary care providers in when and how to self-administer a steroid burst when they become ill or if their PEFR drops by a certain percentage.

Patient Education

Patient education is crucial. As with any chronic, potentially life-threatening disease, the patient should be a partner in the management of asthma. Smoking is forbidden, as is exposure to "side-stream" smoke. Asthmatics should regularly monitor their PEFR values. Many patients have oral steroids at home for use during viral illnesses.

Patients should also be aware of the difference between medications that prevent attacks and those that treat attacks. They should understand the appropriate role of each medication and should take their preventives even when they do not feel any shortness of breath.

PNEUMOTHORAX

Chief Complaint

A 28-year-old man complains that, for the past 2 days, he has had respirophasic (i.e., pleuritic) right-sided chest pain associated with shortness of breath. He smokes a pack of cigarettes each day, sings in a choir on Sundays, and works as a computer programmer. He denies a history of asthma or trauma. He also denies malaise, fever, or symptoms of an upper respiratory infection.

Clinical Manifestations

The patient is tall and slender, alert, and somewhat anxious. Palpation of his chest wall does not reproduce the pain. Careful auscultation suggests decreased breath sounds on the right but does not find wheezes, rales, or ronchi. Placing the stethoscope on his mediastinum, you gently scratch the lateral anterior chest wall on alternate sides, equidistant from the stethoscope. The right side seems louder.

Epidemiologic Factors

Unilateral respirophasic chest pain with dyspnea is the classic presentation of pneumothorax. The incidence of pneumothorax has been variously quoted as 1.7–18 per 100,000; it is significantly more common in males, especially tall and slender young men. Over half of the cases occur in persons younger than 40 years of age. The primary risk factor for persons over 50 is COPD. In all age groups, smoking is the single greatest risk factor, with 80% of pneumothorax cases occurring in smokers (5).

One episode of pneumothorax predisposes to another. Approximately one-third of persons with a history of one episode develop a second episode; and, of those with two episodes of pneumothorax, about half suffer a third (6).

Pneumothorax is classified by etiology as spontaneous or traumatic and by extent of collapse as small, medium, or large. Traumatic pneumothorax implies fairly significant injury and should be evaluated in a hospital. Therefore, it will not be discussed in this chapter.

Spontaneous pneumothorax can be either primary (idiopathic) or secondary. Secondary pneumothorax can be caused by minimal barotrauma, such as that associated with change in ambient air pressure or commercial air travel. Prolonged breath-holding when straining, such as during childbirth, emesis, or lifting sports, or breath-holding combined with noxious gases, such as those from cocaine or marijuana, have frequently been cited as risk factors. Necrotizing infections, such as streptococcal pneumonia or tuberculosis, were the most common etiologic factors for secondary spontaneous pneumothorax until the late 1800s (5). Rupture of weak pulmonary connective tissue (such as in Marfan's syndrome, sarcoidosis, or pulmonary fibrosis) can result in pneumothorax. Occasionally, neoplasms can erode the visceral pleura or an embolism can necrose the pleura, resulting in pneumothorax.

Risk Factors

• Smoking
• Asthma

- Barotrauma
- Positive pressure breathing
- Necrotizing infections
- Tuberculosis
- AIDS (especially in association with *Pneumocystis carinii* pneumonia)

Catamenial pneumothorax, or recurrent pneumothorax associated with menstruation, is exceedingly rare.

Pathophysiology

The basic pathophysiology of pneumothorax is explained by the elastic recoil of pulmonary tissue, which is normally counteracted by the vacuum effect of the close approximation of the moist visceral and parietal pleura. Once this space is violated, either from outside (communicating pneumothorax) or from a pulmonary leak (simple pneumothorax), air enters the pleural space and pulmonary elastic recoil contracts the lung until the tensions balance again.

Occasionally, the break in continuity produces a flap or ball-valve effect that allows air entrance with each inhalation while preventing air escape during exhalation. Air can get in but not out. This ever-increasing volume in the pleural space leads to displacement of the thoracic structure away from the site of injury, compromising both blood return to the heart and air exchange in the undamaged lung. Untreated tension pneumothorax can rapidly become fatal.

Laplace's law explains the increased risk of pneumothorax with hyperinflation states or bullae. If F represents the tension on the wall of a curved surface, D, the diameter, and P, the pressure gradient, then Laplace's law can be written mathematically as $F \propto D \times P$. This equation implies that the larger the diameter of a sphere, the greater the tension on the wall; therefore, the risk of rupture is greater. This simple statement explains why abdominal aortic aneurysms greater than 5 cm in diameter carry an increased risk of rupture, why patients with emphysema are at risk for pneumothorax, and why abscesses drain spontaneously.

Diagnosis

The diagnosis of pneumothorax ultimately is radiographic, but a pneumothorax of 10% or more may be strongly suggested by a number of clinical maneuvers. Generally, breath sounds are decreased on the affected side, and a lack of tactile fremitus exists. Subcutaneous emphysema may be present. The scratch test described above reveals better sound transmission on the involved side; oxygen saturation by pulse oximeter may be unexpectedly low. Arterial blood gases, if assessed, may reveal an increased A-a gradient; and the electrocardiographic findings can mimic acute anterior non–Q-wave MI. Interestingly, the electrocardiogram (ECG) usually corrects if it is obtained in the standing position (7).

A plain chest x-ray is usually sufficient to make the diagnosis of pneumothorax. When it is not, an expiratory or a lateral decubitus film may exaggerate the separation between the chest wall and the lung to demonstrate an otherwise obscure pneumothorax. A pneumothorax of 15% or less is considered small; 15%–60%, moderate; and more than 60%, large.

Tension pneumothorax is the term for a pneumothorax in which air can enter the pleural space with each inspiration but cannot escape with exhalation because of a valve-like opening. The pleural volume builds up, creating pressure that can displace the mediastinum toward the noncollapsed side, which eventually compromises air entry into the "good" lung and finally blood return to the heart and cardiac filling.

Tension pneumothorax should be suspected in the setting of severe respiratory distress with severely diminished or absent breath sounds, hypotension, and bulging neck veins. Deviation of the trachea away from the side of the pneumothorax is a late sign. Patients may present to an office rather than to a hospital. As tension pneumothorax that could progress rapidly to death is easily mitigated, the office practitioner must be aware of the immediate, lifesaving measures described below.

Management

The initial treatment of suspected tension pneumothorax is immediate needle thoracostomy. The method described is optimal, and all the equipment should be available in most offices. However, a simple 18-gauge needle inserted in the second to third intercostal space at the mid-clavicular line and left in place can save a life while equipment is located and emergency services are called.

If no immediate threat to life exists, first assess the degree of dyspnea, the work of breathing, and the adequacy of oxygenation. Confirm the diagnosis radiographically. Treatment is determined by the size of the pneumothorax.

Treatment ranges from observation to needle aspiration to tube thoracostomy. Tension pneumothorax, after initial management with needle thoracostomy, and any bilateral pneumothorax should be treated with tube thoracostomy (8). For moderate to large or increasing pneumothorax, tube thoracostomy (in the hospital) is indicated if respiratory insufficiency is found, regardless of the size of the pneumothorax; if ventilator support is needed; or anytime that air evacuation or transport is contemplated. Additional indications for tube thoracostomy include complete lung collapse, failure of simple aspiration, and underlying lung disease.

Small pneumothorax (see above) can be treated in the office by either observation or needle thoracostomy, with daily radiographs until resolution. Tube thoracostomy becomes necessary if evidence of a continuing air leak remains.

Needle thoracostomy has regained favor since the advent of modern catheter-over-needle IV catheters diminished the risk of further lung injury during pleural space aspiration.

Needle Thoracostomy Equipment

- Buffered local anesthetic, at least 10 mL
- 16-18 g catheter-over-needle
- Three-way stopcock
- 20- to 60-mL Luer-lock–tipped syringe

Needle Thoracostomy Technique

The capacity to diagnose and treat potential complications of needle thoracostomy should be in place before nonemergency needle thoracostomy is attempted. The office should at least have high-flow oxygen, bag-valve-mask equipment, chest radiography, and perhaps the capability to intubate and control the airway if further damage to the lung occurs.

Insert the needle into the second to third intercostal space, mid-clavicular line, on the affected side; remove the needle as soon as the pleural space is penetrated; and aspirate through the stopcock. Empty the syringe of air through the other port. A tension pneumothorax can be converted to an open pneumothorax with a Swan needle; or, in the office setting, a one-way "flutter valve" can be rigged by cutting a flap in the fingertip of an examination glove and attaching it to the hub of the catheter with a rubber band. Tension pneumothorax or aspiration of more than 1 L of air is an indication for tube thoracostomy.

Referral

Surgical referral becomes mandatory if the needle aspiration withdraws more than 3 L, if the pneumothorax is large or recurrent, or if any suspicion of a disease that requires surgical diagnosis or treatment is aroused. Surgical treatment of pneumothorax may include open thoracotomy with resection bullae, wedge resection, oversewing of a continuing air leak, or pleural abrasion or pleurodesis to adhere the visceral to parietal pleura. Pleural resection is currently discouraged because of the risk of making further thoracotomy impossible.

Follow-up

Reexpansion pulmonary edema is a complication that can be prevented by ensuring that no more than 1 L of air is removed at any one time. Even after successful resolution of a pneumothorax, the patient remains at risk for recurrence and should be closely monitored during the first few months following correction.

Patient Education

The most important message in patient education is to advise patients to quit smoking. The risk of recurrent pneumothorax diminishes with cessation of smoking. Underlying pulmonary conditions, such as asthma or COPD, should be meticulously controlled. Advise patients against breath-holding or barotrauma. Counseling for drug addiction may be needed where appropriate. Educate patients about the symptoms of pneumothorax, and instruct them to seek immediate medical care for recurrences.

ACUTE CARDIOGENIC PULMONARY EDEMA

Acute cardiogenic pulmonary edema (APE) is characterized by a strong circadian rhythm, presenting suddenly in the very early morning. Because of the severity of the dyspnea, patients are more likely to present to the emergency department than to the office. However, with recent changes in the treatment of APE, office treatment can be lifesaving and may even obviate the need for intensive care unit (ICU) admission.

Chief Complaint

A 68-year-old woman comes to the office just as you arrive at 7 a.m. As you unlock the door, she becomes visibly shorter of breath as she entreats you to help her. She has a history of CHF, hypertension, and diabetes and has had one previous heart attack.

Clinical Manifestations

Vital signs: Respirations 40/min; blood pressure (BP) 220/110 mm Hg; heart rate (HR) 160 bpm.

Physical examination: The patient is a moderately obese woman who is dyspneic and who is using accessory muscles of respiration. Pale and profusely diaphoretic, she has jugular venous distention to the angle of her jaw and rales three-fourths of the way up her chest. You cannot tell if she has a gallop rhythm because of the noisy chest. She has only 1+ pitting pedal edema.

Epidemiologic Factors

Cardiogenic APE is a fairly common disease of the middle-aged or elderly who have "fallen off the Frank–Starling curve." Most patients have preexisting left ventricular failure (LVF), a disorder of rate or rhythm, or an increased peripheral vascular resistance (afterload). The most common cause for non-cardiogenic pulmonary edema is either an inability to excrete fluids adequately (as with renal failure or insufficiency) or a direct insult to the lungs. Pulmonary insults may be toxic, such as exposure to chlorine gas (e.g., from shaking powdered cleanser into a toilet bowl that has cleaning ammonia in it), or they may result from trauma and sepsis. High-altitude pulmonary edema results from a vicious cycle similar to that of cardiogenic pulmonary edema, which is also initiated by a decrease in PaO_2 and by fluid retention without underlying cardiac pathology. Toxic and high-altitude pulmonary edemas are rare in the office setting and will not be discussed.

Risk Factors

- Hypertension
- Diffuse cardiomyopathy
- Renal insufficiency or end stage renal failure on dialysis
- Chronic hypoxemia
- Acute MI or ischemia
- Coronary artery disease

Pathophysiology

Most patients with APE do not demonstrate an acute fluid overload but rather have fallen over the edge of the Frank–Starling curve as a result of a combination of factors, including the natural circadian fluctuations in physiologic catecholamine levels and the nocturnal nadir of bronchial diameter. Patients at risk for APE are those whose cardiopulmonary compensation ability is precarious at best. Their sudden decompensation results from a combination of ventricular dysfunction and elevated peripheral vascular resistance. A small decrease in cardiac contractility causes vasoconstriction. Capillary pressure rises. When capillary hydrostatic pressure exceeds intraalveolar pressure, fluid leaks into pulmonary alveoli. Fluid in the alveoli decreases the uptake of oxygen, further weakening the cardiac pump. The resulting stress causes a release of catecholamines, which further raises systemic vascular resistance and blood pressure (9).

Previously, medical thought was that acute MI was the most common precipitant for APE, but recent work has shown that the circadian onset of APE precedes that of MI by 4 hours (9,10). On the other hand, if the patient with APE presents in the afternoon hours (when most offices are open), the cause in this patient is more likely to be acute MI than it would be in the patient who presents in the early morning hours (11).

Modern treatment aims to lower peripheral vascular resistance, to improve oxygenation, and to increase intraalveolar pressure rather than to remove body water.

Differential Diagnosis

- Fluid overload from missed dialysis or overhydration resulting from renal failure
- CHF (earlier in the spectrum; may be stable)
- Exacerbation of sarcoidosis or COPD (does not improve with vasodilators)
- Myocardial infarction with cardiogenic shock (enzyme markers and changes on ECG)
- Tuberculosis (abnormal pulmonary x-ray)
- Hypertensive urgency (not associated with pulmonary vascular leakage and fluid)
- Toxin-induced pulmonary edema (etiologic agent different; direct lung damage; more difficult to treat)

- Exacerbation of asthma (less fluid, more bronchoconstriction)
- Massive pulmonary embolism (a difficult diagnosis, but x-ray does not show classic APE)
- Dissecting thoracic aorta (Widened mediastinum is classic but is not always present. Lower extremities may have significantly different blood pressure from upper extremities, or a difference between the two arms may be measured.)

Diagnostic Tests

The diagnosis of APE is primarily clinical. The classic presentation is early-morning onset of severe and rapidly progressive dyspnea, profuse diaphoresis, severe hypertension, and pale or cyanotic skin. The person prefers to sit upright and may push away an oxygen mask "so I can get some air!" The diagnosis can be confirmed by chest x-ray, which shows a classic pattern of cardiomegaly and panlobar infiltrate (a "white-out"). Confirming the diagnosis should not delay the initiation of therapy because the best diagnostic test is the rapid response to appropriate therapy. APE responds as quickly as it starts. However, to exclude some of the above diagnoses, obtaining an ECG and electrolytes panel with creatinine and blood urea nitrogen (BUN) may be wise if the office has access to these tests or if a sample of the patient's blood can be sent immediately to the hospital or nearest laboratory facility.

Management

Modern pharmacologic therapy is based on the reduction of left ventricular (LV) afterload and on an increase in alveolar oxygen and barometric pressures (11). Some measures, such as intubation with positive end-expiratory pressure (PEEP), may be impractical in the average office setting. Therefore, this section focuses on treatments that can be administered in the office, after emergency medical services have been notified. The renal dialysis patient who has missed a treatment can be stabilized in the same way, pending transfer to a dialysis unit (12).

Outmoded treatments abound in the literature. Bloodletting has no place in modern medicine; rotating tourniquets can cause thrombosis and embolism. Morphine increases the risk of intubation and length of ICU stay (13). Although morphine has a beneficial mild vasodilator effect caused by histamine release, concomitant respiratory depression worsens LV function. Although some diuretics reduce systemic resistance, they also increase heart rate and may elevate the pulmonary capillary wedge pressure. Since up to 50% of APE patients are euvolemic, diuresis *per se* is of no benefit to them. Now that the modern pharmacy has developed medications that cause vasodilatation directly, the medical community no longer needs to rely on the beneficial side effects of drugs whose primary results lie elsewhere.

The physiologic office management of APE begins with monitoring physiologic responses while assisting ventilation and initiating treatment.

Administer 100% oxygen, 2–5 sublingual nitroglycerin tablets, and an angiotensin-converting enzyme (ACE) inhibitor (crushed captopril, 25 mg sublingually) (14). Monitor heart rate, blood pressure, and pulse oximetrics. Establish an IV line and call 911. A diuretic is sometimes indicated, but only after vasodilatation has restored renal blood flow.

Treatment should take precedence over establishing an IV line or monitoring. Noninvasive respiratory support via a bag-valve mask raises pulmonary alveolar pressure and decreases the work of breathing, both of which improve cardiac function. While keeping a tight seal, squeeze the bag as the patient begins to inhale; do not hinder exhalation. Switch to 100% oxygen by non-rebreather facemask as soon as the patient maintains a pulse oxygen reading of 98% or better.

The sublingual route is favored for medications because of its ease and speed of administration. Nitrates increase venous capacitance and may reduce peripheral vascular resistance. This decreases blood return to the heart and, thus, pulmonary blood flow and pressure. This, in turn, decreases LV preload. Give 1–5 nitroglycerin tablets (0.4 mg) sublingually at one time. (Moisten the sublingual space, if necessary.) Repeat every 5 minutes until blood pressure and heart rate begin to normalize. Up to 2 inches of nitroglycerine ointment can be used *after* the initial diaphoresis and cutaneous mottling have abated. Aspirin, 81 mg or 325 mg, should also be administered as MI is an important differential diagnosis.

ACE inhibitors reduce pulmonary capillary wedge pressure within 10 minutes, and dyspnea will improve within 15 minutes. They cause relaxation of the left ventricle and peripheral vasodilatation. As peripheral vascular resistance falls, more blood returns to the heart from the pulmonary bed. A 25-mg tablet of captopril can be crushed, moistened, and administered sublingually. It is well absorbed through the mucus membrane. Although this usage is common, if not state-of-the-art, in emergency medicine, the practitioner should note that sublingual captopril is an off-label use. Captopril's peak effect occurs at 30 minutes. Enalapril (Vasotec) is currently the only FDA-approved intravenous ACE inhibitor; the dose is 1.25–2.5 mg (one or two ampules) IV push, but this is much less likely to be available in an office setting.

Referral

Treatment must be initiated as quickly as possible because APE can be fatal within 30–60 minutes from the onset of the first symptoms. Although MI is not the usual precipitant in early-morning APE, an immediate ECG, transport to the hospital, and admission for observation are prudent. Consider echocardiography for the evaluation of myocardial contractility.

Follow-up

Follow-up after hospitalization includes optimizing treatments for any precipitating conditions that may have been found, such as MI or hypertension, and the avoidance of catecholamine mimetics. Although many patients will be maintained on ACE inhibitors upon discharge, ACE inhibitors can cause angioedema (see Chapter 10). Many patients can and should learn to monitor their own blood pressure at home and to keep records of the results. Chronic diuretic therapy can lead to hypotension and electrolyte imbalances.

Patient Education

After an episode of APE, the patient is at increased risk for another episode. Counsel the patient about the importance of compliance with medication and the risks of airplane travel (reduced ambient oxygen pressure), and advise him or her to call for emergency medical services transport if he or she notes rapidly progressing dyspnea or climbing blood pressure. The most appropriate place for a patient with APE is a hospital or emergency department.

PULMONARY EMBOLISM

Occasionally, a patient presents to the office complaining of dyspnea that turns out to be caused by a pulmonary embolism (PE). Since a large PE can rapidly be lethal and a small PE can leave residual pulmonary damage, establishing the diagnosis can be as important as it is difficult. Most current diagnostic and therapeutic modalities are hospital-based, but the suspicion of PE is based on history, physical examination, and simple office tests. Prevention is always better than treatment; prevention of a PE may be lifesaving.

Chief Complaint

A 34-year-old woman complains of shortness of breath with mild respirophasic chest pain. The dyspnea started suddenly on the day after she returned from a visit to the other coast. She takes birth control pills and smokes a pack of cigarettes per day. She has no history of asthma.

Clinical Manifestations

She is tachypneic at 22 breaths per minute and tachycardic at 102 bpm. Heart sounds are regular, with no murmurs. Lungs are clear without any rales or wheezes. She has no swelling of either leg and bilaterally negative Homans' sign. Her pulse oximeter reading is 93% on room air. You consider pneumothorax as a diagnosis; but the scratch test is negative, as is the office chest x-ray. You also suspect a pulmonary embolus, perhaps caused by deep venous thrombosis (DVT) in the pelvis.

Syncope, rather than dyspnea, can be the presenting complaint in PE (15). Pulmonary embolism should be considered in the differential diagnosis of every syncopal event, even in the face of cardiac dysrhythmias and normal pulse oximetry values.

Epidemiologic Factors

The majority of cases of PE are not identified. Approximately 650,000 cases of PE are identified each year in the United States and result in 60,000 deaths. Untreated, PE causes pruned vasculature and pulmonary damage. Thromboembolic disease tends to recur.

Risk Factors

More than 80% of patients with PE have at least one risk factor for venous thrombosis. Virchow's triad of hypercoagulability, venous stasis, and intimal damage holds true today. Many factors, such as smoking, malignancy, estrogen therapy, inflammatory bowel disease, nephrotic syndrome, trauma, COPD, vasculitis, and a variety of inheritable conditions (such as protein C, protein S, or antithrombin III deficiencies), can bring about a hypercoagulable state. Venous stasis results from immobility: prolonged sitting, dehydration during airplane travel, morbid obesity, strokes, or severe cardiac disease (congestive failure). Intimal damage to blood vessels from venipuncture or intravenous drug abuse may precipitate thrombus formation.

The clot that embolizes may or may not be obvious. A negative Homans' sign does not exclude a lower-extremity clot. Clots are common in the pelvic veins and can also be found in the heart itself. The originating clot may be in an upper extremity or in the pelvic abdomen, although 70%–90% of patients with proven PE are eventually found to have a clot in the lower extremity. However, not all eventually demonstrable clots are detectable on physical examination.

Factors predictive of higher mortality from PE include an age of greater than 65 years, male sex, preexisting malignancy, or right ventricular dysfunction.

Pathophysiology

Pulmonary embolization blocks blood flow to a discrete area of the lung. Usually, the vascular tree distal to the clot necrotizes; but the lung tissue itself does not, which creates a permanent ventilation–perfusion mismatch. What little blood does pass through may spend a longer time in contact with the aerated alveoli, but the majority of the blood is shunted through alveoli whose oxygen has already been absorbed, thus resulting in a lower P_{O_2} and a higher P_{CO_2}. The patient compensates by increasing respiratory rate, but this increase is not usually sufficient enough to normalize the arterial blood gases (ABGs).

Diagnosis

Differential Diagnosis

- Pneumothorax (radiograph and scratch test positive)
- Pneumonia (usually with fever and purulent rather than bloody sputum)

- Pneumomediastinum (may be associated with "crunching" heartbeats)
- Aortic dissection (usually more painful; associated with shock, unequal blood pressures)
- Asthma (wheezing is usually present; PEFR should improve after beta agonist therapy)
- Pleurisy (a diagnosis of exclusion)
- Myocardial infarction (look for ECG changes)
- Pericarditis (patients prefer to sit up and lean forward)

Associated illnesses may include emboli to other organs (e.g., brain) and valvular disease.

Diagnostic Tests

The chest x-ray, though helpful for excluding other potential causes of dyspnea, cannot diagnose a PE by itself. The chest x-ray is necessary for proper interpretation of the ventilation–perfusion (V/Q) scan. The chest x-ray is normal in the majority of patients with PE; however, pleural effusions, subsegmental atelectasis, pulmonary infiltrates, or elevated hemidiaphragm may be found. "Hampton's hump," a wedge-shaped opacity representing a pulmonary infarction, is exceedingly rare (16). A normal chest x-ray in a patient with severe dyspnea and hypoxemia without bronchospasm or anatomical cardiac shunt is strongly suggestive of PE.

The V/Q scan remains the initial diagnostic test of choice for nonmassive PE. It must be used in combination with clinical suspicion. Before ordering the V/Q scan, the clinician should make a clinical assessment of the likelihood of an embolism: small, moderate, or large. A low-probability scan together with a low clinical suspicion virtually excludes a PE; a high clinical suspicion with either a moderate- or high-probability scan is sufficient to indicate that treatment should be commenced. An indeterminate scan combined with anything more than very low clinical suspicion suggests the need for additional testing. The results of the scan combined with the level of clinical suspicion can produce a positive predictive value of 96% and a sensitivity of 85%–90%.

The ECG is the most helpful tool for excluding other diagnoses, such as pericarditis or MI. The most common findings in PE include sinus tachycardia and nonspecific ST-T changes. Other classic abnormalities are found in a minority of patients. These include new-onset atrial fibrillation or right heart strain ($S_1Q_3T_3$, right axis deviation).

Tests that are unlikely to be available in the office may be ordered through the hospital laboratory. ABGs, if abnormal, can help; but a normal ABG does not exclude the diagnosis. In more than 25% of patients, the PaO_2 is more than 80 mm Hg, and 10%–15% of patients will have a normal A-a gradient. D-dimer is the degradation product of cross-linked fibrin and is a nonspecific marker for activation of the antithrombosis system. It is elevated in infection,

MI, and metastatic cancer. This test shows promise but has not been sufficiently developed for clinical use.

Echocardiography also is unlikely to be available in a typical office setting. It can detect right ventricular dysfunction and may even be sensitive enough to detect a thrombus in the pulmonary artery. Transesophageal echocardiogram (TEE) is very specific and is better than 90% sensitive for large clots. Additionally, TEE can detect other life-threatening conditions that present as chest pain and dyspnea, such as aortic dissection, cardiac tamponade, and acute valvular lesions. Spiral computed tomography (CT) is perhaps the diagnostic modality of choice in the relatively stable patient, but it too is unavailable in most offices. Regardless of the technology available, PE is foremost a clinical diagnosis requiring vigilance and suspicion. If the diagnosis is suspected, hospitalization should be sought.

Referral

A patient with a large PE should be managed in an ICU, perhaps optimally by an intensivist. The management may require the attention of pulmonary, hematology, and critical care specialists. A thoracic-vascular surgeon may be consulted about the possibility of embolectomy or placement of a vascular (Greenfield) filter to prevent further embolization. The advent of low molecular weight heparins (LMWHs) may eventually lead to office treatment of suspected but small pulmonary emboli.

Management

Medications and interventions in management of pulmonary embolism are as follows:

- Oxygen supplementation
- Heparin
- LMWH
- Thrombolytics
- Coumarin (Coumadin)

Traditionally, PE has been treated with IV heparin followed by oral anticoagulants (17). LMWHs have shortened the time needed in the hospital for IV medication. LMWHs are derived from standard heparin but are more bioavailable, with fewer side effects and a longer half-life, making laboratory monitoring less necessary. Home therapy of DVT with LMWH has comparable outcomes with dramatic cost savings and offers the potential for early discharge of PE patients as well (18).

Thrombolytics have revolutionized the treatment of clots in the heart vessels; they are touted as immediate treatment for acute cerebral thromboembolic events and, theoretically, should be applicable to blocked vessels in the lung. Unfortunately, as the diagnosis of PE is difficult, the definitive diagnosis can seldom be made within the 3-hour window of safe thrombolysis. Thrombolysis for PE is not FDA-approved, and its safe use awaits a more rapid and precise diagnostic test.

Follow-up

Potential problems and complications include pulmonary fibrosis and chronic V/Q mismatches. These, in turn, can reduce exercise tolerance and can predispose the patient to other pulmonary or cardiovascular problems. In addition, the state that caused the initial thrombosis may predispose the patient to other episodes of thromboembolization.

Patient Education

Pulmonary embolism and a propensity to thrombosis is usually a long-term condition. Patients need to be educated about the many ways they can reduce their risk of a thrombotic event. They should keep well hydrated and should avoid smoking and prolonged immobilization. When traveling, they should move their legs and feet often and should take a short walk every hour. An aspirin prior to long car or airplane trips may be helpful. Some patients at high risk may be advised to have filters placed or may be placed on chronic anticoagulant therapy. Others may be advised to use subcutaneous LMWH while traveling or at high altitude.

REFERENCES

1. Teeter JG, Bleecker ER. Relationship between airway obstruction and respiratory symptoms in adult asthmatics. *Chest* 1998;113(2):272.

2. National Institutes of Health. National Asthma Education Program Expert Panel Report: Guidelines for the diagnosis and management of asthma. NIH Publication 91-3642, 1997.

3. National Heart, Lung and Blood Institute. Highlights of the Expert Panel Report 2: Guidelines for the diagnosis and management of asthma. NIH Publication 97-4051, 1997.

4. Alario AJ, Lewander WJ, Dennehy P, et al. The relationship between oxygen saturation and the clinical assessment of acutely wheezing infants and children. *Pediatr Emerg Care* 1995;11(6):331–339.

5. Emerson CP. Pneumothorax: a historical clinical and experimental study. *Johns Hopkins Rep* 1993;11:1.

6. Rusch VW, Girisberg RJ. Chest wall, pleura, lung and mediastinum. In: Schwartz SL, ed. *Principles of surgery*, 3rd ed. New York: McGraw-Hill, 1999:685–687.

7. Rosen P, Barkin RM. *Emergency medicine.* St Louis: Mosby–Year Book, 1992.

8. Vargas J. Pneumothorax. In: Schwartz GR, ed. *Principles and practice of emergency medicine.* Philadelphia: Lippincott Williams & Wilkins, 1999:616–619.

9. Sacchetti AD, Harris RH. Acute cardiogenic pulmonary edema. What's the latest in emergency treatment? *Postgrad Med* 1998;103(2):145–147, 153–154, 160–162 passim.

10. Anigbogu J, Alkuja S, Totten VY, Miller A. Time of onset of acute pulmonary edema. Oral presentation to the AECOM Regional Pulmonary Consortium's Research Conference, May 21, 1996.

11. Kitzis I, Zeltser D, Kassirer M, et al. Circadian rhythm of acute pulmonary edema. *Am J Cardiol* 1999;83(3):448–450.

12. Sacchetti AD, McCabe J, Torres M, Harris RI-I, eds. Management of acute congestive heart failure in renal dialysis patients. *Am J Emerg Med* 1993;11:644–647.

13. Hoffman JR, Reynolds S. Comparison of nitroglycerin, morphine and furosemide in treatment of presumed pre-hospital pulmonary edema. *Chest* 1987;92:586–593

14. Barnett B, Cruzon C. Sublingual captopril in the treatment of acute heart failure. *Curr Ther Res* 1991;49:274.

15. Wolfe TR, Allen TL. Syncope as an emergency department presentation of pulmonary embolism [see comments]. *J Emerg Med* 1998;16(1): 27–31.

16. Tapson VF, Carroll BA, Davidson BL, et al. The diagnostic approach to acute venous thromboembolism: clinical practice guideline. *Am J Respir Crit Care Med* 1999,160(3):1043–1066.

17. Hauer KE. Low-molecular-weight heparin in the treatment of deep venous thrombosis. *West J Med* 1998;169(4):240–244.

18. Kirchmaier CM, Wolf H, Schafer H, Ehlers B, Breddin HK for the Certoparin Study Group. Efficacy of a low molecular weight heparin administered intravenously or subcutaneously in comparison with intravenous unfractionated heparin in the treatment of deep venous thrombosis. *Int Angiol* 1998;17(3):135–145.

Cardiovascular

Paul R. Pfeiffer

ANGINA

Angina is a symptom complex caused by an imbalance in the supply and demand of myocardial oxygen. Angina is associated with a disturbance in myocardial function but not with myocardial necrosis.

Angina can be divided into three major types: stable, variant, and unstable. Stable angina consists of episodic pain that lasts 5–15 minutes; it is usually provoked by exertion and is relieved by rest or nitroglycerin. Variant angina, or Prinzmetal's angina, often occurs at rest and is thought to be caused by coronary vasospasm. Unstable angina has been divided into three presentations by the U.S. Agency for Healthcare Research and Quality (formerly the Agency for Health Care Policy and Research): rest angina, new-onset angina, and accelerating angina. Rest angina is associated with anginal symptoms that occur at rest, that last longer than 20 minutes, and that have occurred within a week of presentation. New-onset angina is angina with onset within 2 months of presentation that occurs with walking one to two blocks or climbing one flight of stairs. Accelerating angina, which occurs more frequently, has a longer duration or begins with less provocation.

Chief Complaint

A 65-year-old man presents with a history of hypertension, diabetes mellitus, and hypertriglyceridemia and complains that this time his typical "angina" is not being helped by nitroglycerin.

A 73-year-old woman arrives at the office for a routine physical examination. She mentions that she feels a pressure (gesturing deep to the precordium) every time she walks to the bird feeder. She states that it always goes away after she sits down.

The first case represents unstable angina; the second case, stable angina.

Clinical Manifestations

Signs and symptoms of angina are numerous (Table 4.1). The family physician should perform a brief, initial evaluation of the cardiac, pulmonary, neurologic, and renal systems. The physical examination is frequently normal. As with most medical conditions, an accurate history may be the single most important step in categorizing a patient's risk. Supine, sitting, and standing

T ABLE 4.1.   Signs and symptoms of angina

- Dyspnea on exertion—may be the only symptom
- Discomfort described with a clenched fist over the sternum (Levine's sign)
- Precordial pressure or heaviness radiating to the back, neck, or arms, brought on by exercise, emotional stress, meals, cold air, or smoking and relieved by rest or nitrates
- Discomfort may radiate to neck, lower jaw, teeth, shoulders, inner aspects of the arms or back
- Diaphoresis from sympathetic discharge; nausea from vagal stimulation
- Decreased exercise tolerance
- Elderly patients and those with diabetes may have atypical presentations

bilateral blood pressures and pulses should be taken in all patients who present to the office with angina. Evaluating patients for severe hypotension (possible ventricular dysfunction) or hypertension (possible catecholamine release precipitating angina) is very important. Cardiac auscultation is useful in evaluating for new murmurs, third and fourth heart sounds, and left ventricular size and function. Inspection of the eyes may reveal a corneal arcus, and examination of the skin may reveal xanthomas. Rales on pulmonary examination suggest mitral regurgitation or left ventricular dysfunction.

Epidemiologic Factors

Angina is thought to be the presenting symptom of coronary artery disease in 38% of men and 61% of women. The actual prevalence is limited by the variable nature of the disease and by the need to diagnose almost entirely on basis of the combination of history, electrocardiographic findings, and risk factors.

Risk Factors

Numerous predisposing factors have been implicated (Table 4.2).

- *Age.* Angina increases linearly with age.
- *Sex.* Angina is diagnosed more often in men between the ages of 40 and 70. After the age of 70, women and men are equally affected.
- *Family history.* Coronary artery disease has genetic implications.

Pathophysiology

Angina results from reduced blood flow to the heart, which is caused by atherosclerosis of the coronary arteries. Four possible causes of reduced coronary flow have been identified (Table 4.3). Coronary thrombosis generally is superimposed. Associated factors include the following:

- Location and severity of the atherosclerotic narrowings in the coronary arterial tree.
- Size of the vascular bed perfused by the narrowed vessel(s).
- Oxygen needs of the poorly perfused myocardium.

T ABLE 4.2.   Risk factors for angina

- Hypercholesterolemia (increased low-density lipoproteins; decreased high-density lipoproteins)
- Hypertension
- Tobacco use
- Diabetes mellitus
- Male sex
- Advanced age
- CAD or family history of premature CAD (onset before age 55)
- Obesity
- Sedentary lifestyle
- Hypertriglyceridemia
- Previous cerebrovascular accident
- Peripheral vascular disease

CAD, coronary artery disease.

- Extent of development of collateral blood vessels.
- Presence, site, and severity of coronary arterial spasm.
- Presence of tissue factors capable of modifying the necrotic process.
- Activity and effect of endogenously released thrombotic and thrombolytic substances.

Diagnosis

Family physicians should remember that the initial diagnosis of angina is based almost entirely on the history, electrocardiographic findings, and risk factors. Despite recent advances in laboratory detection, the history remains imperative in making a prompt, accurate diagnosis. Table 4 4 lists the differential diagnosis of angina.

Diagnostic Tests

Electrocardiography is one of the most important diagnostic tests in the patient with angina. It may show evidence of prior myocardial infarction

T ABLE 4.3.   Possible pathophysiologic causes of angina

- **Progressive coronary obstruction.** Asymptomatic until stenosis causes impaired oxygen supply versus demand.
- **Coronary vasoconstriction.** Caused by cold stimuli, adrenergic input, or cocaine use.
- **Nonocclusive thrombosis on a preexisting plaque.** Likely affects the majority of patients. Preexisting plaque is disrupted, resulting in incomplete coronary occlusion.
- **Coronary inflammation.** New evidence points to inflammation as a possible etiologic factor in atherogenesis and thrombogenesis. *Chlamydia pneumoniae* and *Helicobactor pylori* are thought to be associated with coronary heart disease. C-reactive protein and amyloid A have been found to be predictive of mortality and future cardiac events.

T ABLE 4.4.   Differential diagnosis of angina

• Aortic dissection	• Pericarditis
• Gastritis	• Anxiety/panic disorder
• Cholecystitis	• Myocardial infarction
• Esophagitis	• Pulmonary embolism
• Esophageal spasm	• Aortic stenosis
• Pneumothorax (spontaneous, iatrogenic, and pneumomediastinum)	• Asthma/reactive airway disease
	• Cardiomyopathy
• Costochondritis (Tietze's syndrome)	• Hypertensive emergencies

(MI), or it may show changes during a patient's symptom phase or during treatment. A normal electrocardiogram (ECG) or an unchanged tracing from the baseline does not exclude ischemic causes.

Creatine kinase (CK) rises after an MI. The CK level begins to rise 4–8 hours after the event, peaks in 18–24 hours, and subsides over 3–4 days. The CK level is the most specific indicator for myocardial necrosis but has a 15% false-positive rate.

CK isoenzymes (MM, BB, MB) are identified with skeletal muscle (MM), brain and kidney tissue (BB), and cardiac muscle (MB). This laboratory test is the gold standard for detection of myocardial necrosis. Generally, CK-MB activity exceeds 5% of total CK activity in patients with acute MI.

Troponin is a contractile protein normally not found in serum. Its sensitivity for MI is superior to CK-MB within the first 6 hours for detection of myocardial necrosis.

Complete blood count (CBC) is useful in patients who have suspected anemia.

Basic metabolic profile (BMP) is useful in evaluating renal function, serum glucose, and electrolytes.

Echocardiography, both two-dimensional and M-mode, is useful for evaluating wall motion abnormalities caused by ischemia, overall left ventricular function, and mechanical complications.

Chest x-ray may illustrate alternative causes of chest pain, such as pneumonia, thoracic aneurysms, or pneumothorax.

Management

The treatment goals are rapid identification of patients with acute MI and the exclusion of alternative causes of nonischemic chest pain. Initial management should rest on an assumption that the pain is ischemic in origin. After ambulance personnel have been notified, the family physician should initiate supplemental oxygen via nasal prong cannula, pulse oximetry, and telemetry monitoring, if possible. The physician should also obtain a 12-lead ECG and establish intravenous (IV) access. The patient should be given 81 mg or 325 mg of aspirin and sublingual nitroglycerin every 5 minutes for a total of 3 hours if the chest pain is ongoing, if the blood pressure is stable, and if the clinician suspects the pain to be cardiac in origin.

Referral

If the family physician feels the patient is at high risk (e.g., a person with a history of unstable angina), immediate transportation to the emergency department in an ambulance with advanced cardiac life support (ACLS) capabilities should be obtained. Notification and discussion with the emergency department physician and possibly with a cardiologist, along with prompt communication of the patient's electrocardiography results, history and physical examination findings, and medication list, will expedite treatment.

Follow-up/Prognosis

Follow-up of the patient with angina is determined by the patient's needs. Hospitalization for initiation of IV heparin and any necessary further intervention is indicated in patients with suspected unstable angina.

The most common complications among patients with angina are arrhythmias, cardiac arrest, and congestive heart failure (CHF), all of which are related to ongoing cardiac ischemia. The annual mortality among patients with angina is 3%–4% overall.

Patient Education/Prevention

The family physician should discuss with the patient the risk factors for angina, which include high blood pressure, tobacco use, a high-fat/high-cholesterol diet, lack of regular aerobic exercise, and nonadherence to therapy. Patients should be instructed to follow up with their personal physician and to adhere to lifestyle modifications. They should understand the importance of evaluation in the emergency department for changes in frequency or severity of angina. Educational materials may be obtained by contacting the American Heart Association, 7272 Greenville Avenue, Dallas, TX 75231; (214) 373-6300.

MYOCARDIAL INFARCTION

Acute MI is defined as myocardial necrosis. It results from a sustained and complete reduction of blood flow to a portion of the myocardium and is caused by an acute thrombosis at the site of a disrupted atherosclerotic plaque. It is the end product of untreated unstable angina, and its diagnosis requires two of the following three criteria established by the World Health Organization:

- Clinical history (more than 20 minutes consistent with ischemia).
- Ischemic changes on ECG.
- Positive myocardial isoenzyme testing.

Infarcts can be classified as Q-wave (transmural), which is associated with total coronary obstruction, or non–Q-wave (nontransmural), which is associated with a highly narrowed but patent infarct-related artery. Family physicians must remember that myocardial necrosis is complete 4–6 hours after total occlusion and that coronary flow must remain above 40% of preocclusion levels for myocardium to survive.

Chief Complaint

A 66-year-old man presents with discomfort in the chest, left arm, and jaw. He appears anxious and diaphoretic. He describes the sensation as a "weight" on his chest.

A 71-year-old woman with history of hypertension, hypertriglyceridemia, and diabetes mellitus presents to the office with light-headedness, nausea, chest tightness, and epigastric pressure. The patient is not taking estrogen replacement therapy.

Clinical Manifestations

Signs and symptoms of acute MI are numerous (Table 4.5). As with most medical conditions, an accurate history may be the single most important element in determining a patient's risk. The family physician must categorize a patient's risk as high (acute ischemia or infarction), intermediate (stable angina), or low (nonischemic or noncardiac). Factors that should be considered include the onset, duration, location, pattern of radiation, and intensity or quality of the pain, as well as associated symptoms.

Epidemiologic Factors

In the United States, nearly 1.5 million patients suffer from acute MI annually, and approximately 25% of all deaths result from acute MI.

T ABLE 4.5. Signs and symptoms of acute myocardial infarction

Pain in the arm, back, jaw, neck, chest, epigastrium
Anxiety
Light-headedness, syncope, weakness, pallor
Jugular venous distention
S_4 heart sound
Arrhythmias
Nausea and/or vomiting
Chest tightness or heaviness
Cough, dyspnea, rales, wheezing
Diaphoresis
Hypertension, hypotension
Cannon jugular venous A waves (in the presence of heart block or right ventricular failure)

Risk Factors

The classic epidemiologic risk factors are of limited diagnostic utility in the acute setting (Table 4.6). In this setting, the history and clinical findings are more instructive.

Family History

Premature (earlier than 55 years of age) familial onset of coronary disease puts patients at significant risk for acute MI.

Age

The predominant age of patients with acute MI is over 40 years.

Sex

Between the ages of 40 and 70 years, risk of acute MI is higher among men than women. At 70 years of age and older, men and women are at equal risk.

Pathophysiology

Almost all MIs result from atherosclerosis of the coronary arteries, generally with superimposed coronary thrombosis. Associated factors include the following:

- Location and severity of the atherosclerotic narrowings in the coronary arterial tree.
- Size of the vascular bed perfused by the narrowed vessel(s).

T ABLE 4.6. Risk factors for acute myocardial infarction

Hypercholesterolemia (increased low-density lipoproteins; decreased high-density lipoproteins)
Tobacco use
Diabetes mellitus
Hypertension
Premature (before age 55) familial onset of coronary disease
Sedentary lifestyle
Advanced age
Hypertriglyceridemia
Obesity
Male sex
Previous hypercoagulability
History of cocaine or other sympathomimetic drug use
Psychosocial and behavioral factors
Coronary artery disease
Alcohol
Cerebrovascular accident

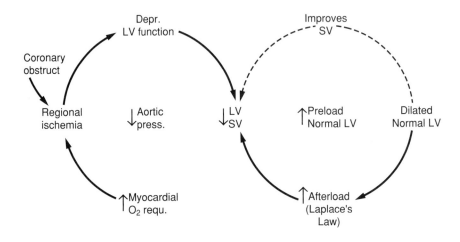

FIGURE 4.1. Changes in circulatory regulation in ischemic heart disease. Aortic press., aortic pressure; Depr. LV function, depressed left ventricular function; O₂ requ., oxygen requirements; SV, stroke volume. Solid lines indicate that the effect is produced or intensified; broken lines indicate that the effect is diminished.

- Oxygen needs of the poorly perfused myocardium.
- Extent of development of collateral blood vessels.
- Presence, site, and severity of coronary arterial spasm.
- Presence of tissue factors capable of modifying the necrotic process.
- Activity and effect of endogenously released thrombotic and thrombolytic substances.

The loss of functioning myocardium is the fundamental pathologic dysfunction. Cessation of blood flow (Fig. 4.1) produces four sequential abnormal muscle contraction patterns (Table 4.7). Unless extension of the infarct occurs, some improvement in wall motion takes place. These improvements are referred to as ventricular remodeling.

Diagnosis

Family physicians should remember that despite recent advances in laboratory detection, the history remains imperative in making a prompt, accurate diagnosis of acute MI. The differential diagnosis is listed in Table 4.8.

T ABLE 4.7. Four sequential abnormal contraction patterns in acute myocardial infarction

Dyssynchrony:	Dissociation in the time course of contraction of adjacent segments of myocardial segments
Hypokinesis:	Reduction in the extent of shortening
Akinesis:	Cessation of shortening
Dyskinesis:	Paradoxical expansion, systolic bulging

T ABLE 4.8. Differential diagnosis of acute myocardial infarction

Unstable angina pectoris:	Use serial ECGs and isoenzyme panel to differentiate. Unstable angina pectoris has a gradual onset, a duration of 5–15 min, and normally, retrosternal location with possible radiation to the neck, jaw, shoulder, and arm with a visceral quality to the pain.
Aortic dissection:	Significant differences in right and left arm blood pressures, hypotension, and unequal or absent pulses differentiate this condition. Aortic dissection has a sudden onset and is associated with constant, severe "tearing" pain with possible interscapular radiation.
Pulmonary embolism:	Sudden onset of chest pain, dyspnea, feeling of impending doom, and respiratory rate greater than 16/min differentiate. Also, there are none of the isoenzyme or electrocardiographic changes that are associated with acute myocardial infarction.
Pericarditis:	History of postural improvement and pleuritic component of pain differentiate.
Esophageal spasm:	Presence of dysphagia usually differentiates. Also, no isoenzyme or electrocardiographic changes associated with acute myocardial infarction are present.

Diagnostic Tests

Creatine kinase (CK). CK rises following infarction. This rise begins 4–8 hours after the event; peaks in 18–24 hours and subsides over 3–4 days. This is the most specific indicator for myocardial necrosis but has a 15% false-positive rate.

CK isoenzymes (MB, BB, MM). MM forms are identified with skeletal muscle, BB in brain and kidneys, and MB in cardiac. Generally, CK-MB activity exceeds 5% of total CK activity in patients with acute MI; specificity is greater than 95%.

Lactic dehydrogenase (LDH). LDH rises above normal values within 24 hours of infarction. The level peaks in 3–6 days and normalizes in 7–10 days.

Troponin. Troponin increases within a few hours and may remain increased for at least 6 days. Half-life is 120 minutes.

Electrocardiography. Physicians must remember that ST-segment elevation is consistent with MI but is a poor predictor of subsequent Q-wave evolution. Serial ECGs are often required in the first 24 hours (Table 4.9).

Echocardiography. Two-dimensional and M-mode echocardiography are useful in evaluating wall motion abnormalities in MI, as well as overall left ventricular function and mechanical complications.

Management

The treatment goals in the patient with acute MI are analgesia, prevention and treatment of electrical and mechanical complications, limitation of infarct size, and protection of viable myocardium. Delay in thrombolytic or invasive treatment is linearly related to increased mortality. Initiating treat-

T ABLE 4.9. Factors predictive of acute ischemia

- Q waves of 1 mm or greater, not previously present, in at least two contiguous leads
- ST-segment changes, either 0.5 mm or more elevation or 1 mm or more depression, in at least two contiguous leads
- T-wave changes, either hyperacuity (>50% of maximum QRS amplitude) or inversion (excluding aVr) in at least two contiguous leads
- New conduction disturbances and/or arrhythmias

ment within the first hour after the onset of symptoms (commonly referred to as the "golden hour") reduces mortality, prevents further myocardial damage, and affords the opportunity to treat cardiac arrest.

If available in the office setting, oxygen via nasal prong cannula should be started; and the patient should be placed on a cardiac monitor while vital signs are obtained and further evaluation is carried out. Nonenteric coated aspirin should be given, provided no contraindication exists. True contraindications include a clear history of severe hypersensitivity, recent (within the past 2 weeks) bleeding ulcerative disease, hemorrhagic stroke, and current active major hemorrhage. A 12-lead resting ECG should be obtained as soon as possible. In some patients, sublingual nitroglycerin is appropriate; the dosage is one tablet every 5 minutes up to a maximum of three tablets.

Referral

If the family physician considers the patient to be at high or intermediate risk, the patient should be transported immediately to an emergency department via an ambulance that has ACLS capabilities. Discussion with the physician in the emergency department and possibly with a cardiologist will expedite treatment. Also, the patient's ECG, history and physical examination findings, and medication list should be communicated. In the patient with acute MI, the most important goal in prehospital care is to reduce the time between infarction and treatment.

Complications/Prognosis

The most common complications noted in the initial 24 hours after acute MI are CHF, arrhythmia, cardiogenic shock, cardiac tamponade, right ven-

T ABLE 4.10. Possible complications of acute myocardial infarction

Death	Congestive heart failure
Cardiac arrest	Cardiogenic shock
Dressler's syndrome	Myocardial rupture
Ventricular septal defect	Left ventricular aneurysm
Mitral regurgitation	Pericarditis
Dysrhythmias	Deep venous thrombosis and pulmonary embolism

T ABLE 4.11. Killip classification of cardiac damage resulting from acute myocardial infarction

Class I	No clinical evidence of shock, mortality <5%
Class II	Mild pulmonary congestion or an isolated S_3 gallop; mortality rate ≤10%
Class III	Pulmonary edema, extensive left ventricular dysfunction; mortality rate ≤30%
Class IV	Hypotension, evidence of shock; mortality >80%

tricular infarction, ventricular rupture, and acute valvular dysfunction (Table 4.10).

The overall mortality rate among patients with acute MI is 10% during the hospital phase; during the 1-year period following the event, another 10% of patients will die. More than 60% of deaths occur within an hour of the onset of the event (Table 4.11).

Patient Education

Education materials may be obtained by contacting the American Heart Association, 7272 Greenville Avenue, Dallas, TX 75231; (214) 373-6300.

HYPERTENSIVE URGENCY/EMERGENCY

Hypertensive urgencies and emergencies require prompt recognition and treatment. Because considerable overlap exists between the two classifications, sometimes a clear distinction can be difficult to establish. A hypertensive emergency, also known as a hypertensive crisis, occurs when an acute elevation of blood pressure causes rapid and progressive end-organ damage. One percent of all patients with hypertension will experience a hypertensive emergency. No predetermined criteria for the level of blood pressure necessary to induce a hypertensive emergency have been established. Evidence of altered organ function, not blood pressure level, is the basis for this diagnosis. Hypertensive urgency, on the other hand, is an elevation of blood pressure to a level that is potentially harmful and is usually sustained at greater than 115 mm Hg diastolic, without signs, symptoms, or other evidence of end-organ dysfunction (Table 4.12). A hypertensive urgency is most often the result of nonadherence to drug therapy.

Chief Complaint

A 42-year-old man presents to the office for routine physical examination. The nurse notes a blood pressure of 240/140 mm Hg. The patient is asymptomatic; he illustrates no evidence of target organ disease during examination.

A 65-year-old man with a known history of progressive aortic dissection presents to the office with a blood pressure of 160/110 mm Hg.

The first case is a hypertensive urgency; the second is a hypertensive emergency.

T ABLE 4.12. Hypertensive emergencies and urgencies

Hypertensive emergencies

Hypertensive encephalopathy

Malignant hypertension (some cases)

Catecholamine excess states

    Pheochromocytoma crisis

    Food or drug interactions (tyramine) with monoamine oxidase inhibitors

Some cases of rebound hypertension following sudden withdrawal of antihypertensive agents (e.g., clonidine [Catapres], methyldopa [Aldomet])

Head trauma

Hypertension following coronary artery bypass

Drug-induced hypertension (some cases)

    Overdose with sympathomimetics or drugs with similar action (e.g., phencyclidine [PCP], lysergic acid diethylamide [LSD], cocaine, phenylpropanolamine [PPA])

Eclampsia or severe hypertension during pregnancy

Postoperative bleeding at vascular suture lines

Severe hypertension in association with acute complications

    Cerebrovascular

        Intracerebral hemorrhage

        Subacute hemorrhage

        Acute atherothrombotic brain infarction (with severe hypertension)

    Cardiac

        Acute aortic dissection

        Acute left ventricular failure with pulmonary edema

        Acute myocardial infarction

        Unstable angina

Hypertensive urgencies

Accelerated and malignant hypertension

Acute glomerulonephritis with severe hypertension

Scleroderma crisis

Acute systemic vasculitis with severe hypertension

Severe epistaxis

Sudden withdrawal of antihypertensive agents

Drug-induced hypertension

    Overdose with sympathomimetic agents (as above)

    Metoclopramide (Reglan)—induced hypertensive crisis

    Interaction between an α-adrenergic agonist and a nonselective β-adrenergic antagonist

Episodic and severe hypertension associated with chronic spinal cord injury

Surgically related hypertension

    Severe hypertension in patients requiring immediate surgery

    Postoperative hypertension

    Severe hypertension after kidney transplantation

Clinical Manifestations

Severe and generalized headache and visual impairment (blurring or variable loss of acuity) are the most common initial symptoms (Table 4.13) of both hypertensive urgency and emergency. The family physician should perform a brief, initial evaluation of the neurologic, cardiac, pulmonary, and renal systems to assess end-organ damage and to rule out secondary causes of hypertension, such as renovascular hypertension or antihypertensive drug withdrawal. The physical examination should include supine, sitting, and standing bilateral blood pressures and pulses, inspection of the abdomen for bruits, a full funduscopic examination for grade 3 or 4 changes, and cardiac auscultation with evaluation of left ventricular size and function.

Hypertensive emergencies include hypertensive encephalopathy (headache, irritability, confusion, and altered mental status caused by cerebrovascular spasm), hypertensive nephropathy (hematuria, proteinuria, and progressive renal dysfunction secondary to arteriolar necrosis and intimal hyperplasia), pulmonary edema, aortic dissection, intracranial hemorrhage, preeclampsia/eclampsia, and MI.

Hypertensive urgencies affect patients with no obvious end-organ damage.

Epidemiologic Factors

Hypertension affects 15%–25% of the adult population in the United States. Fewer than 1% of patients with hypertension will experience a hypertensive emergency.

Risk Factors

Obesity, positive family history, black racial heritage, diabetes, advanced age, and low socioeconomic status are key risk factors. Nonadherence to or withdrawal from certain medications, such as central nervous system depressants and antihypertensive agents, puts patients at risk for hypertensive urgencies and emergencies. Drug use, including ethanol, decongestants, steroids, monoamine oxidase inhibitors (MAOIs), cocaine, amphetamines, and appetite suppressants, also predisposes patients to these crises.

T ABLE 4.13.   Signs and symptoms of hypertensive crisis

Nausea	Stupor
Vomiting	Visual loss
Funduscopic hemorrhages, exudates, and papilledema	Focal deficits
	Seizures
Headache	Coma
Confusion	Renal oliguria and azotemia
Somnolence	Congestive heart failure

Family History

Hypertensive emergencies and urgencies are genetically linked.

Age

These crises affect young or middle-aged patients with known hypertensive disease.

Sex

Males are at greater risk than females.

Race

A higher incidence of hypertensive emergencies is found among blacks than among whites.

Pathophysiology

Whenever blood pressure rises and remains above a critical level, various processes overwhelm the autoregulatory mechanisms, which causes further increases in pressure and vascular damage. Two distinct processes are involved in the pathogenesis. One is functional and allows excessive blood flow and vascular dilatation. The other is structural and manifests as increased permeability, which causes acute edema and damage to the arteriolar wall. Both processes are associated with end-organ hemorrhage and edema caused by the leakage of blood and fluid.

Diagnosis

Initial screening is best done with serial blood pressure measurements, using an appropriately sized cuff (inner rubber bag should be wide enough to cover two-thirds of the length and three-fourths of the circumference of the upper arm or thigh, while leaving the antecubital or popliteal fossa free). Two or more readings should be obtained from both arms. Cardiopulmonary decompensation may best be revealed by examining for a prominent left ventricular impulse, increased jugular venous distention, an S_4 or S_3, orthopnea, cyanosis, dependent edema, and hepatomegaly. Funduscopic changes, such as hemorrhage and papilledema, and changes in the exudate may be seen. Remember that the clinical situation and the presence or absence of end-organ damage, not the blood pressure level alone, constitute the severity of a hypertensive crisis. The differential diagnoses are listed in Table 4.14.

Diagnostic Tests

Laboratory

Urine drug screening in selected patients, serum electrolytes, pregnancy screening where appropriate, blood count, and blood smear for microangio-

T ABLE 4.14. Differential diagnoses of hypertensive crisis

Acute anxiety with hyperventilation syndrome
Encephalitis
Hypercalcemia
Acute left ventricular failure
Cerebrovascular accident
Head injury
Cushing's syndrome
Anxiety
Pregnancy (preeclampsia/eclampsia)
Pheochromocytoma
Serotonin syndrome
Epilepsy
Overdoses and withdrawal from narcotics, amphetamines, etc.
Brain tumor
Subarachnoid hemorrhage

pathic hemolytic anemia or thrombocytopenia can be instructive. Urinalysis may illustrate proteinuria, microscopic hematuria, and glycosuria. Subsequent workup for renal artery stenosis or pheochromocytoma may be appropriate in selected patients.

Imaging

Chest radiographs may show pulmonary edema, evidence of coarctation of the aorta, cardiomegaly, and mediastinal widening consistent with a dissecting aortic aneurysm.

Others

Electrocardiography may reveal ischemia or left ventricular hypertrophy.

Referral

Patients with a hypertensive urgency can be adequately managed by the family physician within a few hours in the outpatient setting.

Patients presenting with evidence of hypertensive emergencies require immediate blood pressure reduction in the intensive care setting. Family physicians may need to orchestrate management with neurologists, cardiologists, pulmonologists, critical care physicians, or ophthalmologists depending on the organ systems involved.

Management

Hypertensive emergencies require immediate inpatient blood pressure reduction to prevent or to limit target-organ disease (Table 4.15). Immediate

T ABLE 4.15. Intravenous therapy for hypertensive emergencies

Drug	Dosage	Onset of action	Duration of action	Adverse effects*	Cautions
Sodium nitroprusside (Nipride)	0.25–10 μg/ kg/min as IV infusion† (maximal dose for 10 min only)	Immediate	1–2 min	Nausea, vomiting, muscle twitching, sweating, thiocyanate and cyanide intoxication	Use with caution with high intracranial pressure or azotemia
Nitroglycerin (Tridil, Nitro-bid IV)	5–100 μg/ min as IV infusion†	2–5 min	3–5 min	Headache, vomiting, methemoglobinemia, tolerance with prolonged use	Use with caution in severe hepatic or renal disease
Enalaprilat (Vasotec)	1.25–5 mg every 6 hr IV	15–30 min	6 hr	Precipitous fall in pressure in high-renin states; response variable	Avoid in acute myocardial infarction
Hydralazine (Apresoline)	10–20 mg IV	10–20 min	3–8 hr	Tachycardia, flushing, headache, vomiting, aggravation of angina	Use with caution in CAD and pulmonary hypertension
Diazoxide (Hyperstat)	50–100 mg IV bolus repeated, or 15–30 mg/ min infusion	2–4 min	6–12 hr	Nausea, flushing, tachycardia, chest pain	Use with care in impaired cerebral or cardiac circulation
Labetalol (Normodyne, Trandate)	20–80 mg IV bolus every 10 min, or 0.5–2.0 mg/ min IV infusion	5–10 min	3–6 hr	Vomiting, scalp tingling, burning in throat, dizziness, nausea, heart block, orthostatic hypotension	Not for use in acute heart failure
Esmolol (Brevibloc)	250–500 μg/ kg/min for 1 min, then 50–100 μg/ kg/min for 4 min; may repeat sequence	1–2 min	10–20 min	Hypotension, nausea	Use with caution with asthma and impaired renal function

continued

T ABLE 4.15 *continued.* Intravenous therapy for hypertensive emergencies

Drug	Dosage	Onset of action	Duration of action	Adverse effects*	Cautions
Verapamil (Calan, Isoptin)	5–10 mg IV bolus over 2 min; 10 mg after 30 min, if initial response is inadequate	3–5 min	30 min	Bradycardia, headache, dizziness, nausea	Avoid in seizure, LV dysfunction; use with caution in impaired renal function

*Hypotension may occur with all agents.

† Requires special delivery system.

CAD, coronary artery disease; IV, intravenous; LV, left ventricular.

Adapted from the Sixth Report of the Joint National Committee on Prevention, Detection, Evaluation, and Treatment of High Blood Pressure. Bethesda, MD: National Institutes of Health, 1997. NIH publication no. 98-4080.

reduction is defined in the Sixth Report of the Joint National Committee (JNC VI) as a 25% drop in blood pressure (mean arterial pressure) within minutes to 2 hours, followed by a goal of near 160/100 mm Hg within 2–6 hours. Immediate clinical situations include acute MI, CHF with evidence of pulmonary edema, intracerebral bleeding, and acute aortic dissection. Clinical situations that require reduction in minutes to hours include pheochromocytoma, hypertensive encephalopathy, and eclampsia. Precipitous decreases in blood pressure should be avoided.

JNC VI suggests reduction in blood pressure within a few hours in patients with hypertensive urgencies (Table 4.16). Initially, using a quiet room and reevaluating should be attempted. Remember to treat the patient, not the numbers. Use of oral or sublingual nifedipine (Adalat, Procardia) in the acute setting has recently fallen out of favor because of evidence that it causes a rapid fall in blood pressure and worsens cardiac and cerebrovascular ischemia.

Follow-up

Once blood pressure control has been obtained, the family physician can begin long-term oral therapy. The patient should be seen for follow-up every 1–2 weeks until adequate control is achieved. If treatment goals have not been met after 3 months, the dosage should be changed; a different class of drug should be tried; or a second drug from another class should be added.

Patient Education

Family physicians should counsel their patients about the importance of adherence to antihypertensive treatment and about the dangers of abruptly stopping medication.

T ABLE 4.16. Oral therapy for hypertensive urgencies

Agent	Dosage	Onset	Comments
Clonidine (Catapres)	100–200 µg initially, followed by 50–100 µg/hr; up to a maximum of 800 µg/d	30–60 min	Drowsiness, dry mouth, withdrawal hypertension, bradycardia
Labetalol (Normodyne, Trandate)	100 mg twice daily; maximum of 2,400 mg/d	1–3 hr	Bronchospasm, postural hypotension
Captopril (Capoten)	25 mg, repeat as required; do not exceed 450 mg/d	15–30 min	Hypotension, renal failure in bilateral renal artery stenosis
Nifedipine (Procardia)	10–20 mg, repeat after 30 min; >180 mg/d not recommended	15–30 min	Rapid, uncontrolled reduction in blood pressure may precipitate circulatory collapse in patients with aortic stenosis

DISSECTION

Aortic dissection is caused by an intimal tear, usually transverse, that provides entry for blood to dissect the media and that may separate the intima from the adventitia. It usually occurs along the right lateral wall of the ascending aorta where the shear stress is high. Two-thirds of cases are located in the proximal 1–5 cm of the ascending aorta. Aortic dissections are classified according to the location of origin (Table 4.17).

Chief Complaint

A 65-year-old man with hypertension presents to the office with an abrupt onset of a "tearing" pain in the anterior chest wall that radiates to the interscapular region and back.

T ABLE 4.17. DeBakey and Stanford classifications of aortic dissection

DeBakey	Stanford	Description of dissection
Type I	Type A	Originates in the aortic root with distal extension
Type II	Type A	Localized in the ascending aorta
Type III	Type B	Occurs distal to the left subclavian artery
Subgroup A		Occurs above the diaphragm
Subgroup B		Occurs below the diaphragm

A 33-year-old man presents with excruciating chest pain and a recent syncopal episode. He has a history of Marfan's syndrome.

Clinical Manifestations

Diagnosis of aortic dissection can be challenging even in the inpatient setting. Clinical clues may include the following:

- Significant differences in right and left arm blood pressures.
- Hypotension (particularly in patients with proximal dissection).
- Diastolic murmurs, indicating new aortic insufficiency.
- Neurologic manifestations (e.g., stroke, paresis, ischemic neuropathy, paraplegia).
- Unequal or absent pulses (Table 4.18).

Syncope is an ominous sign and usually indicates rupture of the ascending aorta into the pericardial space.

Epidemiologic Factors

The incidence of aortic dissection is 5–10 patients per million population per year, or approximately 2,000 cases annually.

Risk Factors

- Hypertension is clearly the major risk factor in aortic dissection.
- Age. Age prominence is dependent on etiologic factors.
- Most common between the sixth and eighth decades.
- Patients with Marfan's syndrome commonly present in the third and fourth decades.
- Sex. Men are affected more often than are women, with a ratio of 3:1.

T ABLE 4.18. Signs and symptoms of aortic dissection

Chest pain
Tearing or ripping feeling
Nausea
Dyspnea
Diaphoresis
Weakness
CVA-like symptoms
Altered mental status
Dysphagia
Orthopnea
Anxiety with premonition of impending death
Limb paresthesias, pain, or weakness
Horner's syndrome

CVA, cerebrovascular accident.

Pathophysiology

Death is usually secondary to rupture and tamponade. Approximately 60% of intimal tears occur in the proximal ascending aorta. The remainder are found between the origin of the left subclavian artery and ligamentum arteriosum: 20% in the descending aorta, 10% in the aortic arch, and 10% in the abdominal aorta. Cystic medionecrosis is seen in patients with defects in elastin and connective tissue organization (e.g., Marfan's syndrome, Ehlers–Danlos syndrome).

Diagnosis

Clinical presentation can be challenging. Typically, the patient is an elderly man with known hypertension who presents with excruciating pain of sudden onset in the anterior chest or back. The patient's description of the discomfort as a "ripping" or "tearing" sensation is classic. The differential diagnoses are listed in Table 4.19.

Diagnostic Tests

Retrograde aortography is the gold standard for confirming the presence of an aortic dissection. Disadvantages of this procedure include its invasiveness and contrast requirements.

Chest x-ray may illustrate widening of the superior mediastinum, left pleural effusion, enlargement of the aortic knob, double density of the descending aorta, cardiomegaly, rightward displacement of the trachea, separation of more than 5 mm of intimal calcification from outer aortic contour, and irregular aortic contour.

T ABLE 4.19. Differential diagnoses of aortic dissection

Aortic regurgitation
Pericarditis
Cardiac tamponade
Myocardial infarction
Hypertensive emergency
Thoracic outlet syndrome
Aortic stenosis
Gastroenteritis
Myocarditis
Pulmonary embolism
Myopathies
Shock (cardiogenic, hemorrhagic, or hypovolemic)
Peripheral vascular injuries

Electrocardiography may illustrate nonspecific ST-T changes, electrical alternans with associated tamponade, and left ventricular hypertrophy.

Echocardiography may illustrate dilated aortic root, oscillating intimal flap, pericardial effusion, and increased aortic posterior or anterior wall thickening.

Combined transthoracic and transesophageal echocardiography with color flow Doppler imaging may provide an alternative to retrograde aortography because it is minimally invasive, may be performed at the bedside, and does not require contrast media.

Contrast-enhanced computed tomography (CT) scanning may reveal dissections not shown on aortography, but the sensitivity and specificity of this procedure is not as high as that of aortography or echocardiography.

Magnetic resonance imaging (MRI) also provides detailed images of the aorta, but its value in critically ill patients is limited because of the time required and because the patient is inaccessible, in the event that emergency treatment is necessary, during the procedure. It has the advantages of being noninvasive, of not requiring IV contrast, and of a high diagnostic accuracy.

Management/Referral

If available in the office setting, oxygen via nasal prong cannula should be started; and the patient should be placed on a cardiac monitor until emergency transportation to an appropriate facility arrives. Obtaining a 12-lead resting ECG as soon as possible is crucial to exclude other causes, such as acute MI. Notification and discussion with the emergency department physician, and possibly a vascular surgeon, and prompt communication of the patient's medication list, electrocardiography results, and history and physical examination findings will expedite treatment.

Follow-up

The family physician can improve the survival rate among patients with cardiac dissection through appropriate long-term blood pressure control and close periodic surveillance. Long-term therapy consists of administration of beta blockers plus other antihypertensive agents, such as angiotensin-converting enzyme inhibitors or calcium antagonists.

Patients should be seen 1 month after the initial episode and then should be reevaluated at 3-month intervals for the first year and at every 6 months for the next 2 years. At each 3-month visit, CT scanning with contrast or MRI should be used to detect propagation. After this, follow-up visits may be conducted yearly. Systolic pressure should be maintained at 120 mm Hg or below.

The mortality rate in patients who do not receive treatment is 20% within 24 hours, 60% within 2 weeks, and approximately 90% within 3 months. Hospital survival is estimated at 70% in those who are treated both medically and surgically. Risk of redissection is 13% at 5 years and 23% at 10 years.

Cardiac tamponade, aortic valvular insufficiency, progressive aortic enlargement, redissection, and localized saccular aneurysms are possible complications.

Patient Education

Patients should be educated about modifying risk factors, which include hypertension, tobacco use, elevated blood cholesterol and triglyceride levels, and physical inactivity. After being discharged from the hospital, patients should plan to remain off work for 6-8 weeks.

Diet

Patients should be encouraged to eat properly even if they have a poor appetite. They should remember that the body has a great deal of healing to do after surgery. Discussion with a dietitian is encouraged.

Incision Care

Patients will have a chest incision. They should be assured that some soreness, itching, redness, or numbness at the incision site for the first few weeks after surgery is normal. Use of lotions or powder around incision areas should be avoided until the areas have healed completely. A sensation of movement in the sternum is normal for about 6 weeks.

Emotions

Patients may mention having strange and, often, repetitive dreams. They may feel "let down" or depressed, and they report being tearful and "crying for no reason." Patients should be counseled that these reactions are not uncommon.

Exercise

Patients should follow a walking plan, which is typically outlined after surgery by the vascular surgeon. Patients should exercise briefly several times each day, increasing their workout time by 1-2 minutes each time as long as they are comfortable. Patients should be aware that, when they first get home, even simple routines, such as personal grooming, can be tiring. Patients should be told to avoid the following activities for the first 6 weeks after surgery:

- Repetitive work.
- Unnecessary lifting, pushing, pulling, straining, or other activities during which breath-holding is common.
- Lifting anything heavier than 10-20 pounds.
- Climbing stairs (during the first 1-2 weeks, limit to once or twice daily).

- Vigorous activity in extreme temperatures and/or humidity.
- Alcohol use.

REFERENCES

1. Furberg CD, Psaty BM, Meyer JV. Nifedipine: dose related increase in mortality in patients with coronary heart disease. *Circulation* 1995;92: 1326-1331.

2. Hamm CW, Ravkilde J, Gerhardt W. Prognostic value of serum troponin T in unstable angina. *N Engl J Med* 1992;327:146-150.

3. Hamm CW, Heeschen C, Goldman B. Benefit of abciximab in patients with refractory unstable angina in relation to serum troponin T levels. *N Engl J Med* 1999;340:1623-1629.

4. Wu HB, Abbas SA, Green S. Prognostic value of cardiac troponin T in angina pectoris. *Am J Cardiol* 1995;76:970-972.

5. Hjemdagl P, Eriksson S, Held C. Prognosis of patients with stable angina pectoris on antianginal therapy. *Am J Cardiol* 1996;77(Suppl):6D-15D.

6. Braunwald E, ed. *Heart disease: A textbook of cardiovascular medicine*, 4th ed. Philadelphia: WB Saunders, 1992.

7. Hoekenga D, Abrams J. Rational medical therapy for stable angina pectoris. *Am J Med* 1984;76:309.

8. Braunwald E. Unstable angina: an etiologic approach to management. *Circulation* 1998;98:2219-2222.

9. Theroux P, Fuster V. Acute coronary syndromes: unstable angina and non-Q-wave myocardial infarction. *Circulation* 1998;97:1195-1206.

10. Braunwald E, Califf R, Cannon C, et al. Redefining medical treatment in the management of unstable angina. *Am J Med* 2000;108:41-53.

11. Green LA, Yates JF. Influence of pseudodiagnostic information on the evaluation of ischemic heart disease. *Ann Emerg Med* 1995;25: 451-457.

12. Braunwald E, Mark DB, Jones RH, et al. Unstable angina: diagnosis and management. clinical practice guideline no. 10. AHCPR publication no. 94-0602. Rockville, MD: Agency for Health Care Policy and Research and the National Heart, Lung and Blood Institute, Public Health Service, U.S. Department of Health and Human Services, 1994.

13. Jones EB, Robinson DJ. Unstable angina: year 2000 update. Multi-modal strategies for reducing mortality, urgent revascularization, and adverse cardiovascular events. *Emerg Med Rep* 2000;21(10).

14. Lavie CJ, Gersh BJ. Acute myocardial infarction: initial manifestations, management, and prognosis. *Mayo Clin Proc* 1990;65:531-548.

15. Stack LB, Morgan JA, Hedges JR, Joseph AJ. Advances in the use of ancillary diagnostic testing in the emergency department evaluation of chest pain. *Emerg Med Clin North Am* 1995;13:713-733.

16. AIMS Trial Study Group. Effect of intravenous APSAC on mortality after acute myocardial infarction: preliminary report of a placebo-controlled clinical trial. *Lancet* 1988;1(8585):545-549.

17. The GUSTO investigators. An international randomized trial comparing four thrombolytic strategies for acute myocardial infarction. *N Engl J Med* 1993;329:673-682.

18. Fuster V. Mechanisms leading to myocardial infarction: insights from studies of vascular biology. *Circulation* 1994;90:2126-2146.

19. Pearson T, Criqui M, Luepker R, et al., eds. *Primer in preventive cardiology.* Dallas: American Heart Association, 1994.

20. Zalenski RJ, McCarren M, Roberts R, et al. An evaluation of a chest pain diagnostic protocol to exclude acute cardiac ischemia in the emergency department. *Arch Intern Med* 1997;157:1085-1091.

21. Nichol G, Walls R, Goldman L, et al. A critical pathway for management of patients with acute chest pain who are at low risk for myocardial ischemia: recommendations and potential impact. *Ann Intern Med* 1997; 127:996-1005.

22. Litwack K. Practical points in the differential diagnosis of chest pain. *J Perianes Nurs* 1997;12:363-368.

23. Murata GH. Evaluating chest pain in the emergency department. *West J Med* 1993;159:61-68.

24. Froelicher VF, Quaglietti S.*Handbook of ambulatory cardiology.* Philadelphia: Lippincott-Raven Publishers; 1997.

25. Lee TH, Cook EF, Weisberg M, et al. Acute chest pain in the emergency room. Identification and examination of low-risk patients. *Arch Intern Med* 1985;145:65-69.

26. Guidelines for the early management of patients with acute myocardial infarction. A report of the American College of Cardiology/American Heart Association Task Force on Assessment of Diagnostic and Therapeutic Cardiovascular Procedures (Subcommittee to Develop Guidelines for the Early Management of Patients with Acute Myocardial Infarction). *J Am Coll Cardiol* 1990;16:249-292.

27. Falk E, Shah PK, Fuster V. Coronary plaque disruption. *Circulation* 1995; 92:657-671.

28. Lange RA, Hillis LD. Immediate angioplasty for acute myocardial infarction [Editorial]. *N Engl J Med* 1993;328:726-728.

29. Tierney WM, Roth BJ, Psaty B, et al. Predictors of myocardial infarction in emergency room patients. *Crit Care Med* 1985;13:526-531.

30. Weaver WD. Time to thrombolytic treatment: factors affecting delay and their influence on outcome. *J Am Coll Cardiol* 1995;25(7 suppl):3S-9S.

31. Gifford RW Jr. Management of the hypertensive crisis. *JAMA* 1991;266: 829-835.

32. Vidt DG. Current management of hypertensive emergencies. In: Henning RJ, Grenvik A, eds. *Critical care cardiology*. New York: Churchill Livingstone; 1989:137-168.

33. Kaplan NM. Hypertensive emergencies and urgencies. In: NM Kaplan, ed. *Clinical hypertension*. Baltimore: Williams & Wilkins, 1990:268-822.

34. Price DW. The hypertensive patient in family practice. *J Am Board Fam Pract* 1994; 7:403-416.

35. Grossman E, Ironi AN, Messerli FN. Comparative tolerability profile of hypertensive crisis treatments. *Drug Saf* 1998;19(2):99-122.

36. Strauss FG, Franklin SS, Lewin AJ, Maxwell MH. Withdrawal of antihypertensive therapy. *JAMA* 1977;238:1734-1736.

37. Anderson RJ, Hart GR, Crumpler CP, et al. Oral clonidine loading in hypertensive urgencies. *JAMA* 1981;246:848-850.

38. Calhoun DA, Oparil S. Treatment of hypertensive crisis. *N Engl J Med* 1990;323:1177-1183.

39. Kaplan NM. Management of hypertensive emergencies. *Lancet* 1994; 344:1335-1338.

40. McKindley DS, Boucher BA. Advances in pharmacotherapy: treatment of hypertensive crisis. *J Clin Pharm Ther* 1994;19:163-180.

41. Ferguson R, Vlasses P. Hypertensive emergencies and urgencies. *JAMA* 1986;255:1607-1613.

42. Ledingham J. Management of hypertensive crisis. *Hypertension* 1983; Suppl III: 114-118.

43. McRae R, Liebson P. Hypertensive crisis. *Med Clin N Am* 1986;70: 749-767.

44. Murphy C. Hypertensive urgencies. *Emerg Med Clin N Am* 1995;13: 973-1007.

45. Ram C. Management of hypertensive emergencies: changing therapeutic options. *Am Heart J* 1991;122:356-363.

46. Izzo JL Jr, Black HR, Vidt DG. Emergencies and urgencies: management. *Hypertens Prim Am Heart Assoc* 1993;E22:338-341.

47. Murphy C. Hypertensive emergencies. *Emerg Med Clin N Am* 1995;13 (4):973-1007.

48. Panacek E. Controlling hypertensive emergencies: strategies for prompt, effective therapeutic intervention. *Emerg Med Rep* 1992;13:53-61.

49. Wheat MW Jr. Acute dissection of the aorta. *Cardiovasc Clin* 1987;17: 241–262.

50. Asfoura JY, Vidt DG. Acute aortic dissection. *Chest* 1991;99:724–728.

51. DeSanctis RW, Doroghazi RM, Austen WG, Buckley MJ. Aortic dissection. *N Engl J Med* 1987;317:1060–1067.

52. Crawford ES. The diagnosis and management of aortic dissection. *JAMA* 1990;264:2537–2541.

53. DeBakey ME, Cooley DA, Creech O Jr. Surgical consideration of dissecting aneurysm of the aorta. *Ann Surg* 1955;142:586–612.

54. Nienaber CA, Von Kodilitsch Y, Nicolas V, et al. The diagnosis of thoracic aortic dissection by noninvasive imaging procedures. *N Engl J Med* 1993;328:81–90.

55. Ballal RS, Nanda NC, Gatewood R, et al. Usefulness of transesophageal echocardiography in assessment of aortic dissection. *Circulation* 1991;84:1903-1940.

56. Doroghazi RM, Slater EE, DeSanctis RW, et al. Long-term survival of patients with treated aortic dissection. *J Am Coll Cardiol* 1984;3:1026-1034.

57. DeBakey M, McCollum CH, Crawford ES, et al. Dissection and dissecting aneurysms of the aortic: tzwenty-year followup of five hundred twenty-seven patients treated surgically. *Surgery* 1982;92:1118–1134.

58. Sarasin F, Gaspoz J, Junod A, et al. Detecting acute thoracic aortic dissection in the emergency department: time constraints and the choice of the optimal diagnostic test. *Ann Emerg Med* 1996;28(3):278–288.

59. Chen K, Varon J, Wenker OC, et al. Acute thoracic aortic dissection: the basics. *J Emerg Med* 1997;15(6):859–867.

60. Hagan PG, Nienaber CA, Isselbacher EM. The International Registry of Acute Aortic Dissection (IRAD): new insights into an old disease. *JAMA* 2000;283:897–903.

CHAPTER 5

....

Endocrinologic

Richard B. Birrer

DIABETES MELLITUS

Diabetes mellitus, a common diagnosis, affects 6% of the American population: 8% of adults, 1.3% of children, and up to 25% of the elderly. The incidence and prevalence of the disease are increasing annually. Individuals with type 1 diabetes require insulin therapy. Unless management is intensive or "tight," the blood glucose of most patients is "hectic," swinging up or down 200–300 mg/dL daily. Therefore, hyper- and hypoglycemia are frequently occurring complications. Individuals with type 2 diabetes mellitus develop these complications less commonly; their insulin resistance serves as a buffer against such extremes.

Pathophysiology

The elevated blood sugar present in the patient with diabetes mellitus primarily leads to hyperlipidemia, damage to the endothelium of small vessels (secondary to increased extracellular matrix production and nonenzymatic protein glycosylation), leukocyte dysfunction, and an increase in sorbitol. Over time, the former leads to atherosclerotic cardiovascular disease that with hypertension and sorbitol-enhanced platelet aggregation synergistically results in the well-recognized complications of cerebral, myocardial, and extremity infarction. Increased amounts of sorbitol also lead to early formation of cataracts. Neuropathy, retinopathy, and glomerulosclerosis develop from the microvascular disease and the elevated levels of sorbitol. Infections follow leukocyte dysfunction and are often worsened by the associated microvascular disease.

Complications

The remainder of this chapter will discuss glycemic urgencies and emergencies. Some of these, such as hypo- and hyperglycemia, can be caused by lack of patient persistence (compliance), neglect, or poor care. However, because these conditions can also result from undiagnosed diabetes, medication complications, or underlying comorbid states, the family physician must carefully evaluate the patient and agressively treat not only the glycemic disorder but also any underlying state.

Hypoglycemia

Blood glucose is the main energy source of the nervous system. Significant brain damage and death can occur from prolonged severe hypoglycemia. Hypoglycemia is defined as a fall in blood glucose concentration to a level that elicits symptoms secondary to glucose deprivation in the central nervous system (generally accepted as less than 50 mg/dL).

CHIEF COMPLAINT

Symptoms are highly variable and range from a feeling of being "off" or "funny" to "having the jitters" to weakness, inattentiveness, and unresponsiveness. The patient actually may be brought in to the office because a family member or caretaker is concerned or has witnessed a seizure, accident, or fall.

CLINICAL MANIFESTATIONS

Although the most common presentation of hypoglycemia is neurologic and mental dysfunction, clinical manifestations vary widely (1). The actual level of blood glucose that causes symptoms is highly individual and is influenced by factors such as weight, gender, age, dietary history, emotional state, physical activity, and comorbid disease. Individuals with plasma glucose levels of 35 mg/dL or lower may be asymptomatic, whereas other individuals who may be symptomatic have glucose levels within the "normal" range. Often, no symptoms are reported because the hypoglycemia occurs at night when the patient is asleep. A patient's perception of hypoglycemia may be blunted by medications and changes in his or her sense of well-being. Generally, the intensity of the counterregulatory response and associated adrenergic symptoms is proportional to the depth of the fall in serum glucose level, rather than the rate.

Unsuspected hypoglycemia can masquerade as a psychiatric, neurologic, or cardiovascular disorder. Symptoms and signs of the hypoglycemic syndrome have two components: sympathetic and central nervous system. The typical sympathetic presentation includes complaints of palpitations, sweating, nervousness, anxiety, irritability, tremor, hunger, lethargy, weakness, pallor, or nausea. Nocturnal hypoglycemia is suggested by a history of nightmares, nocturnal sweating, morning nausea or abdominal distress, general sluggishness, changed personality, or impaired memory. Such complaints may be blunted or absent in persons with neuropathies, particularly in the setting of diabetes, or in those taking sympathetic blocking agents, although diaphoresis is common and may be the only adrenergic symptom in the patient taking a nonselective beta-blocking agent (2).

Neurologically, headache, dizziness, difficulty speaking, and blurred vision may be present (3). In addition, hemiplegia associated with extensor plantar responses lasting for a few hours to a few days, coma, seizures, and cerebral infarction (right more than left) have been well described in adults, adolescents, and children (4). These effects are abrupt but reversible. Cardiopulmonary arrest has been reported. Urticaria, facial flushing, and orthopedic trauma (posterior shoulder dislocation) are associated nonclassical findings.

Hypoglycemia that follows the feeding state occurs within 6 hours of the glucose load following a normal fasting serum glucose level. Symptoms usually occur several hours after eating, particularly in the late morning or late afternoon. Symptoms of early type 2 diabetes are usually mild and brief, lasting 15–20 minutes; and the family history of diabetes is positive. Postgastrectomy hypoglycemia is not the same as the "dumping syndrome." The latter is due to rapid dilutions of hyperosmolar material in the jejunum that produce symptoms of nausea, weakness, pallor, epigastric discomfort, dizziness, palpitations, and diarrhea. The symptoms usually occur within 10 minutes after a meal, subside within 1 hour, and do not result from hypoglycemia. The patient with idiopathic hypoglycemia is typically a healthy young adult with no underlying cause of hypoglycemia. Weakness, lightheadedness, tremors, sweating, confusion, anxiety, and numbness are commonly reported. A clue to fasting or postabsorptive hypoglycemia may be that the patient is difficult to arouse in the morning, following an overnight fast; or the patient may simply lapse into a coma. Symptoms of an insulinoma include a combination of palpitations, blurred vision, diplopia, sweating, weakness, seizures (12% of the time), and confusion or abnormal behavioral patterns (80% of patients, with 50% lapsing into coma or experiencing amnesia for the duration of the hypoglycemic episode). Symptoms may be aggravated by exercise and may occur at irregular intervals but are more common in the late afternoon (before dinner) or in the early morning (before breakfast). Symptoms may vary in duration and, in the majority of cases, may be alleviated by eating. Regrettably, the interval between the initial onset of the hypoglycemic symptoms and the diagnosis of insulinoma is, on average, 19 months; but it may be years. Hypoglycemia may be profound and cerebral function may be significantly depressed in patients with other neoplasms that cause fasting hypoglycemia. Mass and weight loss are often present.

The clinical recognition of nocturnal hypoglycemia is often difficult. Long-acting insulin preparations taken once daily are typical culprits. Findings of depression, lethargy, nightmares, night sweats, morning headaches, seizures, hepatomegaly due to glycogen accumulation, enuresis, polyuria, polyphagia, weight gain, mood swings, and frequent episodes of rapidly developing ketosis are suggestive of an insulin overdose. Occasionally, medical personnel and diabetic patients or their caretakers may surreptitiously administer insulin or an oral hypoglycemic drug to induce hypoglycemia and simulate organic disease. Such individuals usually are emotionally unstable, exhibit erratic patterns of hypoglycemia, and deny drug misuse even when directly confronted.

EPIDEMIOLOGIC FACTORS

Type 1 diabetes mellitus is the most common cause of hypoglycemia, but hypoglycemia may occasionally be severe in type 2 diabetes. The risk of hypoglycemia is highest in the most tightly controlled patients, particularly children and adolescents, in whom the incidence of hypoglycemia is 18%-60%. More than 90% of emergency department hypoglycemia patients are there as a result of excessive insulin administration. About 10% require treatment, and of those, more than 60% are admitted. Three to seven percent of deaths of patients with type 1 diabetes are due to hypoglycemia. Hypoglycemia caused by long-acting oral antidiabetic agents (Table 5.1) tends to be more refractory to treatment and usually necessitates admission with a dextrose drip (4).

Most cases of *drug-induced* hypoglycemia during the first 2 years of life are caused by salicylates; alcohol is the most common cause in patients 3-10 years of age; for patients 11-30 years of age, 60%-70% of all comas are secondary to insulin or sulfonylurea administration, with half of these occurring

T ABLE 5.1. Pharmacologic causes of hypoglycemia

Angiotensin-converting enzyme inhibitors	Kerola (Herbs)
Acetaminophen	Lithium
Alcohols	Manganese
Amphetamine	Mebendazole (Vermox)
Aspirin	Monoamine oxidase inhibitors
Beta blockers	Nonsteroidal antiinflammatory drugs
Butyrophenones	Onion extract
Calcium	Orphenadrine (Norgesic)
Chloramphenicol	Oxytetracycline (Terramycin)
Clofibrate (Atromid)	Pentamidine (Pentam)
Clotrimazole	Phenylbutazone
Cocaine	Phenothiazines
Dextropropoxyphene	Pyridoxine
Dicumarol	Quinine
Disopyramide (Norpace)	Salicylates
Ethylenediaminetetraacetate	Sublactam/ampicillin
Halofenate	Sulfa drugs
Haloperidol (Haldol)	Tetracyclines
Hypoglycin (Akee Nut)	Theophylline

in nondiabetic young females attempting suicide; between the ages of 30 and 50, alcohol alone or in combination with insulin is a common cause of hypoglycemic coma; and after 60 years, the sulfonylureas are more likely culprits (5–7).

RISK FACTORS

An inverse correlation between the level of glycosylated hemoglobin (HbA$_{1C}$) and the incidence and severity of hypoglycemia has been found. A 36% higher risk exists for each 1% decrease in the HbA$_{1C}$. Individuals with no residual C-peptide are at higher risk than are those who have elevated levels of C-peptide. The Diabetes Control and Complications Trial (DCCT) data indicate that the occurrence of severe hypoglycemic comas is approximately three times higher in patients receiving intensive therapy. Additional risk factors in the pediatric population include undiagnosed child abuse and a high central nervous system to lean mass ratio. The former is supported by evidence of starvation or drug side effect. A crash office delivery should be managed for potential neonatal hypoglycemia.

Additional risk factors include the history of prior hypoglycemic episodes, alcohol use, missed meals or snacks, increased activity, increased disease duration, younger age, and male sex. Up to one-third of these individuals will present either in a coma or with a neurologic abnormality, such as a seizure. Finally, the use of human recombinant insulin has several potential negative effects. Because it provides tighter control and causes fewer adrenergic side effects, patients who use it typically have difficulty recognizing hypoglycemia; and when they do, it tends to be later rather than sooner. The diagnosis of factitious hypoglycemia is more difficult because human insulin is less immunogenic.

The elderly are also at risk for hypoglycemia secondary to medications for associated diabetes, abuse, high central nervous system to lean tissue mass ratio, and significant comorbid states that require hospitalization or that impair functional capacity, resulting in inadequate nutrition (8). The sulfonylureas and sulfonamide drugs are specifically associated with hypoglycemia, and they may blunt the patients' perception of hypoglycemic symptoms, thus increasing risk (5,6). All sulfonylureas (Table 5.1) stimulate the release of insulin from the pancreas with a subsequent decrease in hepatic glucose output. Drug-induced hypoglycemic reactions, whether deliberate or accidental, are often prolonged, profound, and life-threatening. Recurrent hypoglycemic reactions induced by oral hypoglycemic drugs can produce encephalopathy. The concomitant administration of alcohol, salicylates, sulfonamides, coumarin derivatives, and phenylbutazone can potentiate the hypoglycemic effects of the sulfonylureas. Chlorpropamide (Diabinese) is responsible for most cases of hypoglycemia occurring during normal food intake with intact renal function and at ordinary dosages. Hypoglycemia following disopyramide administration has been known to develop in elderly patients who are poorly nourished and have mild abnormalities in glucose homeostasis.

Malnourished chronic alcoholics often develop alcohol-induced hypo-glycemia, although spree drinkers or occasional drinkers who have missed a meal or two may also experience this problem. Several cases have been reported of febrile children who, when treated with continuous sponging using rubbing alcohol, have developed severe alcohol intoxication and hypo-glycemic coma (7). The presentation is usually coma or semicoma 2–10 hours after alcohol ingestion with associated hypothermia, tachypnea, and alcohol fetor. The absence of an odor of alcohol does not rule out alcohol as a cause of the hypoglycemia or coma. Most patients are unresponsive except to deep-pain stimulation. Seizures are particularly common in children. Lab-oratory findings include hypoglycemia, elevated blood alcohol level, mild aci-dosis, and ketonuria without glucosuria.

Hypoglycemia secondary to salicylate overdosage should be considered in any child with coma, cardiovascular collapse, and convulsions. In adults, sal-icylate-related hypoglycemia most often follows aspirin administration in conjunction with other compounds that lower the levels of glucose. In chil-dren, consider oil of wintergreen. β-Adrenergic blockers, particularly pro-pranolol (Inderal), in diabetic patients with angina and hypertension can pre-cipitate hypoglycemia. Lastly, patients receiving hyperalimentation or hemodialysis may develop hypoglycemia following the sudden cessation of a high-concentration glucose infusion.

Although the end result is hypoglycemia, two major types are found: postabsorptive and postprandial (Table 5.2). Hypoglycemia resulting from either may occur spontaneously, whereas induced causes are commonly associated with postabsorptive hypoglycemia.

The recognition of *fasting* or *postabsorptive* hypoglycemia is very impor-tant because the condition often reflects serious underlying organic disease and may be spontaneous. Because the hypoglycemia may develop slowly (5–6 hours after a meal), the signs of hyperepinephrinemia may not be seen. Most patients with the disorder develop low glucose levels during a 24-hour fast. Occasionally, a 72-hour fast is required to establish or to rule out this diagnosis. Hospitalization may be required for complete evaluation.

Insulinomas produce hypoglycemia in the fasting and fed states. Women in their 40s to 70s characteristically develop insulinomas. Because of the sub-tle nature of the disorder, patients may be misdiagnosed as having stroke, brain tumor, epilepsy, narcolepsy, psychosis, anxiety/hysteria state, or even a Stokes–Adams attack.

Virtually every histopathologic neoplasm has been associated with fast-ing hypoglycemia (Table 5.3). Such tumors are often unsuspected and are discovered during systemic evaluation of a patient with fasting hypo-glycemia. Men are more commonly diagnosed with large hepatic carcino-mas than women (4:1). These tumors are associated with a rapidly fatal

T ABLE 5.2.   Types of hypoglycemia

Postabsorptive (fasting)
  Glucose underproduction
    Hormone deficiencies
      Glucagons
      Catecholamines
      Adrenal insufficiency
      Hypopituitarism
    Enzyme defects
    Substrate deficiencies
      Late pregnancy
      Severe malnutrition
      Ketotic hypoglycemia of infancy
    Drugs
    Severe disease
      Hepatic
      Renal
      Sepsis
      Hypothermia
  Glucose overutilization
    Normal insulin levels
      Tumors
      Enzyme deficiencies
      Cachexia
      Systemic carnitine deficiency
    Hyperinsulinism
      Insulinoma
      Exogenous insulin
      Drugs
      Shock
      Sepsis
      Immune disease
Postprandial (fed, reactive)
  Alimentary hyperinsulinemia
  Congenital deficiencies
    Fructose intolerance
    Galactosemia
  Early diabetes
  Leucine insensitivity
  Idiopathic (functional)

T ABLE 5.3. Tumors associated with fasting hypoglycemia

- Mesenchymal tumors of nonpancreatic origin (most common): fibrosarcomas, mesotheliomas, thoracic and retroperitoneal tumors
- Endothelial and epithelial tumors of the breast, ovary, kidney, lung, and gastrointestinal tract (adrenocortical and hepatic carcinomas and carcinoids)

outcome (1–6 months), with hypoglycemia occurring as a terminal or preterminal event. The pathogenesis of tumors with associated hypoglycemia may involve secretion of substances with insulin-like biological activity, the increased utilization of glucose by the tumor, decreased gluconeogenesis from the depletion of substrates and general cachexia, depression of glucagon secretion inactivity, or liver impairment due to metastasis or tumor products.

A number of endocrine-related diseases can produce spontaneous fasting hypoglycemia (Table 5.4). Secondary adrenal insufficiency (hypopituitarism) is more common and severe because of concomitant deficiencies of growth hormone and glucocorticoid.

Functional impairment or destruction of 80%–85% or more of the liver may result in hypoglycemia due to impaired gluconeogenesis and glycogenolysis. Severe pathologic processes due to Reye's syndrome, severe passive congestion, acute viral hepatitis, and acute hepatic necrosis have been implicated. Whereas liver metastases usually do not produce hypoglycemia, involvement of large portions of the liver may do so. Chronic liver disease is rarely a cause of hypoglycemia. Patients with hepatic failure sufficient to cause hypoglycemia are often in a coma, which may be missed if the coma is assumed to be caused by hepatic encephalopathy.

Hypoglycemia has been reported in association with terminal leukemia and following heavy exercise (>90 minutes) when liver glycogen stores are depleted and the rate of glucose production fails to keep pace with the rate of glucose use. The latter condition has been referred to as "bonking." Occasionally, starvation-related hypoglycemia may be seen. The patient is usually a child with kwashiorkor or an adult with anorexia nervosa. *Fasting and fed* autoimmune hypoglycemia resulting from antiinsulin antibodies in patients

T ABLE 5.4. Endocrine-related causes of hypoglycemia

- Deficiencies of glucagon, glucocorticoids, and growth hormone
- Adrenal insufficiency
- Hypothyroidism (especially when severe enough to cause myxedema coma)

not known to have received insulin injections has been documented in several case reports. Hypoglycemia often occurs in the face of overwhelming sepsis in elderly patients and infants with underlying renal and liver disease. The association between severe lactic acidosis and chronic renal failure in diabetic and nondiabetic patients that leads to spontaneous fasting hypoglycemia has been well documented.

The most common cause of induced hypoglycemia is drugs, particularly sulfonylureas, alcohol, and salicylates (Table 5.1). Sulfonamides, such as trimethoprim-sulfamethoxazole (Bactrim), can produce hypoglycemia. Comorbid states (e.g., renal or hepatic disease) and restricted carbohydrate intake increase the risk and severity of drug-induced hypoglycemia.

The most common cause of hypoglycemia seen in the emergent or urgent situation is an insulin reaction in a diabetic patient. The risk of such a reaction is directly related to the severity of the diabetes, with the least production of endogenous insulin creating the widest variation in blood glucose levels. If such patients are taking a nonselective β-adrenergic antagonist, they are at increased risk of severe prolonged hypoglycemic reactions. Gastroparesis, anxiety, exercise, a late meal, inadequate carbohydrates, alcohol ingestion, insulin dosage error, erratic absorption of insulin from subcutaneous sites, and overtreatment with insulin may precipitate hypoglycemia in an insulin-dependent diabetic patient.

Postprandial hypoglycemia, which is spontaneous, follows the fed state and is also called fed or reactive hypoglycemia. There are three major causes of postprandial hypoglycemia: *early diabetes, alimentary hypoglycemia*, and *idiopathic hypoglycemia*. An early manifestation of type 2 diabetes is spontaneous hypoglycemia 3–5 hours after a meal, presumably due to delayed release of insulin with subsequent excessive insulin secretion in response to the initial hyperglycemia.

Following partial or total gastrectomy, pyloroplasty, or gastrojejunostomy, 5%–10% of patients may develop symptomatic *alimentary* hypoglycemia 1–3 hours after a meal. Rapid gastric emptying and an exaggerated insulin response appear to be the causes. A correlation between peak insulin levels and hypoglycemia does exist. Rarely, alimentary hypoglycemia has occurred in the absence of gastrointestinal surgery. Such patients appear to have rapid glucose absorption or release of gut factors that stimulate insulin secretion due to a gut defect.

Diagnosed far more often than is justified, *idiopathic* or *functional* hypoglycemia is probably rare and may simply reflect a transition in intermediary metabolism between the fed and fasting state, usually occurring 2–4 hours after a meal or with minor deprivation of food, such as a missed meal (Table 5.5). Many experts question the diagnosis, and several investigations have documented a poor correlation between symptoms and blood glucose levels.

T ABLE 5.5. American Diabetes Association criteria for idiopathic hypoglycemia

- Documented low blood sugar in conjunction with the particular symptoms about which the patient complains.
- Relief of symptoms by the ingestion of food or sugar.

DIAGNOSTIC TESTS

The office detection and evaluation of hypoglycemia are limited. They include a history and physical examination, an electrocardiogram (ECG), and random serum glucose determination as the main investigative tools. Funduscopic examination for diabetic-associated papilledema and retinopathy is essential. Tachycardia, hypertension, arrhythmias, cardiac ischemia, and an altered mental status may be identified. Lastly, no findings may be present.

The serum glucose should be determined in all patients who have coma; seizures; disturbed sensorium; an unexplained motor vehicle accident; smell of alcohol; an undefinable "funny" smell; or a potential for drug overdose, depression, or suicide and in all diabetic patients with clinically significant complaints. Unfortunately, the fasting early morning blood glucose level may be normal in spite of nocturnal hypoglycemia or may even be elevated (Somogyi phenomenon), leading to an increase in insulin dosage and a worsening of symptoms.

The identification of a low blood sugar by a glucose reagent strip usually differentiates between coma associated with hypoglycemia and hyperglycemic ketoacidosis with coma. The older "dextro-sticks" are less accurate and may give a false low reading. Certainly, hypoglycemic patients will benefit from dextrose, and patients with ketoacidosis will not be unduly harmed by it.

The glucose tolerance test (GTT) is no longer used to confirm the diagnosis of postprandial spontaneous hypoglycemia. The 5-hour test has poor specificity and shows as many as 50% of patients as hypoglycemic.

Diagnosis of insulinomas is made by confirmation of hypoglycemia and hyperinsulinemia at the time of spontaneous symptoms. A prolonged fast up to 72 hours may be required to provoke the hypoglycemia, although 75%–90% of patients develop it before 24 hours of fasting. The differential diagnosis should include surreptitious self-administration of insulin. Immunoreactive C-peptide levels are low with exogenously administered insulin but are proportionally elevated if an endogenous secretory mechanism is intact. In addition, the presence of insulin antibodies suggests self-administration of insulin, although antibodies may not be detectable before 6 weeks to 2 months of exogenous insulin administration.

A blood test for sulfonylureas should be ordered if surreptitious insulin use is suspected. The more potent second-generation agents may not exhibit very high plasma levels. Insulin antibodies will be elevated in someone who has administered insulin for 6–8 weeks. Obtain C-peptide levels if insulin antibodies are not detected or if a diabetic patient is suspected of having factitious hypoglycemia. The level is low if the source of insulin is exogenous and high in cases of endogenous hyperinsulinemia.

All ill women in the third trimester of pregnancy should have a blood glucose determination. The convergence of hemolysis, elevated liver enzyme levels, and low platelet count occurring in association with preeclampsia (HELLP syndrome) has been documented to cause hypoglycemia.

DIAGNOSIS

Anxiety, drug withdrawal, and other physiologic states, such as lactose intolerance, acute cholelithiasis, and the dumping syndrome, are important considerations in evaluating a patient for hypoglycemia.

REFERRAL

Refractory hypoglycemia of unknown origin that necessitates prolonged complex treatment (more than glucose) requires further evaluation.

MANAGEMENT

The outpatient treatment of a conscious patient suffering from hypoglycemia consists of self-administration of oral glucose (Table 5.6). Patients with coma of unknown cause or diabetic adults in coma should be given immediate (over 1–3 minutes) 50 mL of 50% glucose IV bolus after blood has been obtained for appropriate studies (e.g., serum glucose, drug levels, C-peptide, antiinsulin antibodies, insulin, etc.). Even if a blood sugar level is not immediately available and the patient turns out to have diabetic ketoacido-

T ABLE 5.6. Common sources of 20 g of D-glucose

Food	Amount
Apple juice (1 cup)	12.0 fl. oz.
Banana	6.4 oz (1 large or 2 small)
Coke (nondietetic) (12 oz.)	13.3 fl. oz.
Gelatin (sweetened with sugar)	6.4 oz.
Ginger ale (Fanta) (12 oz.)	15.5 fl. oz.
Hershey milk chocolate bar (1.45 oz.)	2.5 oz.
Kool Aid (with sugar) (1 cup)	13.4 fl. oz.
Orange juice (1 cup)	12.0 fl. oz.
Orange soda (Fanta) (12 oz.)	10.0 fl. oz.
Tang (orange with sugar) (1 cup)	10.0 fl. oz.

sis, the extra glucose will not be harmful. If hypoglycemia is confirmed, a follow-up infusion of 5%, 10%, or 20% glucose solution should be started and maintained for at least 4–6 hours. The duration of treatment should be dictated by the underlying cause of hypoglycemia because early discontinuation may result in recurring hypoglycemia. Fructose should not be substituted for glucose because it is a low-calorie sugar that does not cross the blood–brain barrier effectively. The infusion should run at such a rate that the blood glucose level, monitored every 2–3 hours, is maintained at or above 100 mg/dL. The glucose infusion can be stopped once a persistent hyperglycemia is present and is maintained by slow administration of 5% glucose. The patient should be instructed to continue oral carbohydrate intake and to return if any symptoms of hypoglycemia recur.

If the first liter of glucose solution fails to establish or to maintain an elevated glucose level, the patient should be transported to the nearest emergency department. Glucagon (freshly mixed in buffer) administered intramuscularly or subcutaneously in 0.5- to 2-mg doses and 100 mg of hydrocortisone per liter is appropriate. The effect of glucagon will be noted in 10–20 minutes, and the injection may be repeated twice. If given intravenously, a continuous infusion should be used because of the compound's short half-life. It is not effective in the treatment of *alcohol-induced* or *starvation* hypoglycemia because glycogen stores are depleted. Also, there may be delayed absorption of simultaneously ingested carbohydrates because the drug tends to cause gastric atony associated with nausea. IV glucose is usually sufficient to correct the *alcohol-associated* hypoglycemia.

Because the half-life of chlorpropamide in serum is 36 hours, with 3–5 days required for complete elimination from the body, hypoglycemia is often very prolonged and may be refractory to treatment by IV glucose alone. This is particularly true in nondiabetic patients (e.g., intentional overdoses) in whom insulin release mechanisms are intact because the infusion of glucose stimulates insulin release and further lowering of the blood glucose level may occur. Diazoxide (300 mg slow IV fusion over 30 minutes every 4 hours) has been successful in raising the blood sugar to supranormal levels without causing hypotension. All patients with *sulfonylurea-induced* hypoglycemia require hospitalization, observation, and treatment.

The treatment of *alimentary* hypoglycemia focuses on minimizing insulin release by decreasing the amount of ingested carbohydrates. A long-term, high-protein, low-carbohydrate diet is appropriate for patients with *idiopathic* hyperglycemia.

Whereas definitive treatment for insulinoma is surgical excision, which tends to be curative in most cases, frequent feedings of slowly absorbable forms of carbohydrates (e.g., pasta, fresh fruit, whole-grain bread) are indicated. Consideration should be given to the use of diazoxide (Hyperstat IV), which directly inhibits the release of insulin by the β cells. Thiazides often need to be added to counteract the edema secondary to sodium retention.

The treatment for nonresectable neoplasms that cause hypoglycemia includes debulking and oral or IV glucose replacement.

Starvation hypoglycemia may be severe and can be refractory to therapy due to the failure of glucogenesis from fat or protein depletion or because of normally increased cellular glucose consumption. Hospital admission for an infusion of lactated Ringer's solution containing hydrocortisone and 20% dextrose is necessary.

A late-evening carbohydrate snack and a reduction of insulin dosage to avoid hypoglycemia are appropriate management of the Somogyi phenomenon. Adjustment of the evening dose of intermediate- or long-acting insulin to provide additional coverage in the early morning hours is appropriate for the dawn phenomenon and insulin waning. Inappropriate treatment could result from the attribution of early-morning hyperglycemia to the wrong cause (e.g., comorbid condition).

FOLLOW-UP/PROGNOSIS

Office observation utilizing serial examinations, while somewhat arbitrary, should last for at least 3-6 hours while the patient is receiving treatment. Patients with hypoglycemia caused by nutritional deficit, alcohol, or "regular" insulin excess that is responsive to office intervention can go home after they have been stabilized. Hospitalization for observation should be considered for any patient who is not fully recovered an hour after normoglycemia is restored, who has required a 10% dextrose infusion as emergency therapy, or for whom a cause has not been identified. Usually such patients usually have been using intermediate- or long-acting insulins or first- or second-generation sulfonylurea oral hypoglycemic agents.

PATIENT EDUCATION/PREVENTION

The prevention of hypoglycemic reactions in insulin-dependent diabetics is essential; however, less than one-third of all hypoglycemic episodes are symptomatic (9). Anticipatory guidance for diabetic patients is summarized in Table 5.7. The best offense against hypoglycemia is the patient's ability to recognize its symptoms and to avoid a full-blown episode by the oral ingestion of carbohydrates. A source of carbohydrates (at least 10-15 g) should be carried with the patient at all times. Remind patients that the time frame required for the blood glucose level to rise after ingestion and for symptoms to resolve may be 10-20 minutes. Many diabetic patients miss or fail to recognize the early warning cues. Patients with long-standing type 1 diabetes and those with strict glycemic control are less likely to experience any symptoms and therefore are more likely to slip quietly into coma in response to glucose deprivation. Family physicians must identify and advise such diabetic patients, particularly those who drive motor vehi-

T ABLE 5.7. Techniques for prevention of hypoglycemia

- Educate patient and family/friends concerning signs, symptoms, causes, and treatment.
- Instruct on regular self-monitoring of blood glucose.
- Prescribe identification card or medical identification bracelet.
- Provide repeated reviews and updates, including reading material and written instructions.
- Institute periodic nocturnal (3 a.m.) blood glucose level monitoring.
- Review sick-day management protocols.
- Remind patient to assess medication carefully and regularly, nutrition, and exercise programs with appropriate adjustments.
- Provide positive feedback for good judgment.

cles and who are prone to hypoglycemic reactions. Up to one-third of type 1 diabetics who drive will have severe or frequent hypoglycemia in the preceding 6 months of regular driving. Less than 25% of hypoglycemic drivers realize that they are impaired (10). One-third of these patients will be involved in a driving accident. In addition to educating these patients directly about unexpected hypoglycemic reactions, physicians should advise self-monitoring of blood glucose level just before driving and at 1- to 2-hour intervals during long drives. The patient should maintain a blood glucose level above 100 mg/dL, carry an easily available source of sugar, and travel with an informed person who can administer the sugar if necessary. All medications that may cause or potentiate hypoglycemic reactions, particularly alcohol, should be avoided.

Children and adolescents who are being maintained with tight glycemic control regimens should be assessed carefully, with parental guidance for adverse nocturnal hypoglycemia events that are not clinically recognizable. The absolute avoidance of any hypoglycemia (particularly nocturnal) by setting higher glycemic control targets (120–200 mg/dL) for 1–2 months is usually associated with a return of the patient's ability to sense hypoglycemia. Individuals who have had repeated significant episodes of hypoglycemia should be considered for the insulin lispro, which reduces the incidence of hypoglycemia, improves postprandial control, and enhances compliance (11).

The elderly, particularly those who are hospitalized or in a nursing home, who have a significant amount of comorbid disease burden and who may not be diabetic at all, should be monitored carefully for complicating hypoglycemia. Lastly, for patients undergoing office procedures, particularly those requiring conscious sedation, glucose monitoring before and at least every 2 hours after the procedure, with more frequent monitoring in more heavily sedated and high-risk patients, is highly recommended.

REFERENCES

1. Birrer RB. The many facets of hypoglycemia. *Emerg Med* 2000;32(3): 63-77.

2. Hoeldtkerd RD, Boden GO. Epinephrine secretion, hypoglycemia unawareness, and diabetic autonomic neuropathy. *Ann Intern Med* 1994;120:56-127.

3. Field JB. Hypoglycemia. *Endocrinol Metab Clin N Am* 1989;18 (3):27-43.

4. Hepburn DA, Deary IJ, Frier BM, et al. Symptoms of acute insulin-induced hypoglycemia in infants with and without IDDM. A factor analysis approach. *Diabetes Care* 1991;14:949-957.

5. Klonoff DC, Barrett BJ, Nolte MS, et al. Hypoglycemia following inadvertent and factitious sulfonylurea overdosages. *Diabetes Care* 1995;18(4): 563-567.

6. Gerrich JE. Oral hypoglycemia agents. *N Engl J Med* 1989;321: 1231-1245.

7. Ernst AA, Jones K, Nick TG, Sanchez J. Ethanol ingestion and related hypoglycemia in a pediatric and adolescent emergency department population. *Acad Emerg Med* 1996; 3(1):46-49.

8. Teo SK, Ee CH. Hypoglycemia in the elderly. *Singapore Med J* 1997;38 (10): 432-434.

9. Campbell PJ, Gerrich JE. Mechansims for prevention, development and reversal of hypoglycemia. *Adv Intern Med* 1988;33:205-300.

10. Cox DJ, Gonder-Frederick LA, Kovatchev BP. Progressive hypoglycemias—impact on driving simulation performance: occurrence, awareness and correction. *Diabetes Care* 2000;23:163-170.

11. Campbell RK, Campbell LK, White JR. Insulin lispro: its role in the treatment of diabetes mellitus. *Ann Pharmacother* 1996;30(11): 1263-1271.

Hyperglycemia

DIABETIC KETOACIDOSIS

Diabetic ketoacidosis (DKA) is defined by hyperglycemia (blood sugar > 250 mg/dL), acidosis (< 7.35 arterial pH or 7.30 venous pH), and ketonemia or ketonuria (12. DKA is a life-threatening metabolic disorder that is the end result of a relative or absolute lack of insulin. Although it may be triggered by severe physiologic stress, including infarction, pregnancy, infection, or insulin omission, failure to recognize the emergency nature of DKA or its severity is the leading cause of death in patients with diabetes. Fluid deficits are large, electrolyte shifts are massive, and frequently, an underlying serious illness is present.

Chief Complaint

Most patients complain of nonspecific discomfort unless they are comatose or severely obtunded.

Clinical Manifestations

Generalized weakness, fatigue, nausea, and recent weight loss are characteristic. Dehydration and thirst result from vomiting, hyperglycemia, hyperpnea (Kussmaul's respirations), and ketonuria. The dehydration is usually hypotonic. Check for fetor diabeticorum. Carefully evaluate all body systems for complications (skin: poor turgor/tenting; head-ears-eyes-nose-throat: signs of *Mucor, Candida, Aspergillus*, longitudinal tongue furrowing in the elderly, or depressed anterior fontanelle in infants; pulmonary: pneumonia; neurologic: meningitis). Unless the patient is in shock, the blood pressure and heart rate are usually elevated secondary to hypovolemic stress. Hypotension suggests more than 10% dehydration. Patients with severe DKA are often at the limits of their respiratory compensation. Even a small ventilatory compromise can lead to a rapidly fatal outcome. Although the patient's temperature is usually normal or decreased in DKA, sepsis is not necessarily ruled out. Less common symptoms include abdominal, retrosternal, or cervical pain; dyspnea; and dysphonia. Ileus is not an uncommon finding, although subcutaneous emphysema and pneumomediastinum are rare.

Risk Factors

The major risk factors are newly diagnosed diabetes (17%-25%), failure to take insulin (15%-41%), infection (28%-35%), medical illness (10%), miscellaneous (10%-20%), and unknown (2%-25%). Medical illnesses include cerebral and myocardial infarction, pulmonary embolus, and pancreatitis. Trauma, alcoholism, and steroids are examples of miscellaneous factors. Substance abuse and poor insulin compliance are important risk factors. Fundamentally, unless a precipitating illness or a similar form of physiologic stress exists, the occurrence of DKA in patients with established type 2 diabetes represents a failure of patient education. In the presence of one or more obvious causes, one should never assume that other hidden etiologic events for decompensated hypoglycemia do not exist.

Epidemiologic Factors

The incidence of DKA is 14 per 100,000 person-years. Although the incidence is two cases of DKA for every 100 type 1 diabetic patient, a higher incidence is found among younger patients, with 1%-3% occurring in children younger than 1 year (13). Between 50% and 60% of children with new-onset type 1 dia-

T ABLE 5.8. Characteristics of insulin-dependent (type 1) and non–insulin-dependent (type 2) diabetes mellitus

Characteristic	Type 1	Type 2
Prevalence among diabetic patients	10%–20%	80%–90%
Age at diagnosis	Usually <30 yr	Usually >40 yr
Associated obesity	No	Very common
Concurrence in identical twins	<50%	>90%
Specific HLA-D antigen association	Yes	No
Islet cell antibodies present at time of diagnosis	Yes	No
Islet pathologic finding	Isleitis; selective loss of most β cells	Smaller normal appearing islets; amyloid (i.e., amylin) deposition common
Endogenous insulin secretion	Extremely low to undetectable	Normal to high
Insulin resistance	Usually absent	Usually present
Propensity to ketoacidosis requiring insulin for control	Yes	No
Responsive to sulfonylureas or metformin HCl (Glucophage)	No	Yes

HLA-D, human leukocyte antigen D.

betes develop DKA (14). The general admission rate is 14.3 per 1,000 diabetic patients; 8%–28% of all diabetics (average = 19%) are primarily admitted for DKA. In patients with type 2 diabetes, the rates of DKA are 5%–10% of those for patients with type 1 (Table 5.8). The mortality of DKA averages 2%–5%, with higher rates in developing countries (6%–24%) and in certain patient subgroups, such as the elderly (70%–75%) and children (5%–10%). A total of 70% of diabetes-related deaths occur in children with DKA.

Pathophysiology

See Fig. 5.1.

Diagnosis

The differential diagnoses of DKA include hypoglycemia; hyperosmolar, hyperglycemic nonketotic coma (HHNC); postictal states; abdominal emergencies; salicylate, chloral hydrate, and cyanide overdoses; lactic acidosis; uremia; and alcoholic ketoacidosis (ethanol, isopropyl, methanol, ethylene glycol, and paraldehyde derivatives). Starvation and glucose-6-phosphate dehydrogenase (G-6-PD) deficiency can rarely resemble DKA clinically. With the exception of HHNC, the majority of patients with these conditions present with euglycemia or hypoglycemia.

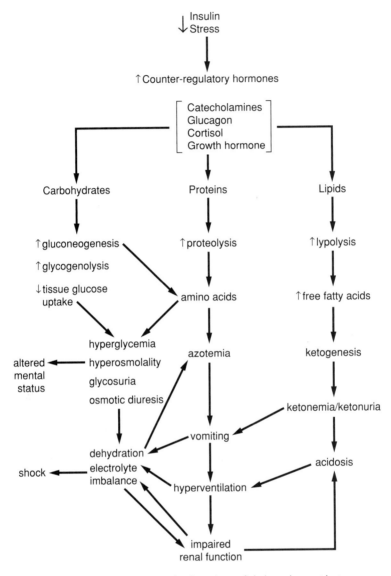

FIGURE 5.1. Pathophysiology of diabetic ketoacidosis.

Diagnostic Tests

Very few (1%) patients with DKA have a normal blood glucose level. The elevation of the blood sugar usually ranges from simple glucose intolerance to frank decompensated hyperglycemia. Similarly, the mental status of a patient with unrecognized DKA can range from normal to comatose. The coma is secondary to hyperosmolarity, not acidosis. The potassium level may be normal secondary to acidosis. The deficit is approximately 5 mmol/kg. The potassium deficit is usually greater in patients with newly diagnosed diabetes than in those with established disease because polyuria has been present for a longer period before the patient was admitted. Additional laboratory findings include hyperosmolarity, hyperlipidemia, electrolyte disturbances, and acidosis. Serum sodium may be spuriously low secondary to osmolar dilution by glucose and the sodium-free lipid fraction. The deficit is usually 10 mmol/kg. Dehydration elevates the blood urea nitrogen (BUN), amylase, albumin, lactate dehydrogenase (LDH), and creatine phosphokinase (CPK). Fractionate the CPK if myocardial pathology is found. The creatinine is often falsely elevated secondary to autoanalyzer methodology interference from ketones present in the serum. Liver enzymes also may be increased due to fatty infiltration. Leukocytosis (<20,000 neutrophilia) can occur as a result of demargination, stress, and dehydration. Sepsis is suggested in the presence of bands. There is usually an anion gap acidosis (>18 mEq/L). Ketones (acetoacetate, acetone, β-hydroxybutyrate) are elevated. Nitroprusside-based tests are unreliable in assessing the true level of serum ketones because they do not detect β-hydroxybutyrate and only weakly detect acetone. If the nitroprusside test is positive, one can safely assume that DKA is present and that the principle ketone is acetoacetate. Ketone production is responsible for the acidosis.

Referral

All patients with suspected DKA (i.e., appropriate clinical manifestations and markedly elevated blood sugar in association with glucosuria and ketonuria) should be referred to the emergency department (ED) for treatment and evaluation for admission. Consultation with an endocrinologist should also be sought for patients with new-onset type 1 diabetes and for those with pregnancy, persistent hyperglycemia, recurrent acidosis, and complicating cerebral edema.

Management

Restoring perfusion through rehydration, stopping ketogenesis by insulinization, correcting electrolyte losses, and avoiding complications are the mainstays in management of DKA (15-17). Most patients with DKA require admission to an observation or step-down unit. Particularly severe cases, in which the patient is younger than 2 years of age or older than 60 years, require admission to the intensive care unit. Outpatient therapy can be considered if the initial pH (determined in the ED) is greater than 7.25 and HCO$_3$ is more than 20 mEq/L, if oral fluids are tolerated, if symptoms resolve in the ED, if no precipitating factor requires hospitalization, and if a reliable caretaker is available. A 0.5- to 1-L infusion of 0.9% normal saline should be given over 2 hours while an expeditious admission is planned. If available, regular insulin at a dosage of 0.1 unit/kg can be given by IV bolus. Bicarbonate should not be given. Fluids alone improve hyperglycemia, hypertonicity, and acidemia secondary to a decrease in counterregulatory hormones and increased renal perfusion. Subcutaneous insulin is not absorbed in severely dehydrated patients, resulting in decreased serum insulin, accelerated ketone formation, and rapid acidosis development. If available, a nasogastric tube is recommended for persistent vomiting, gastric dilation, or coma. Chemical gastritis often produces occult blood. Bear in mind that insulin administration in hypotensive patients who are severely hyperglycemic can lead to vascular collapse. Although many significant management variations are found among specialties with respect to the use of bicarbonate, insulin, fluids, and electrolytes, unanimous agreement that the administration of fluids as soon as possible is the mainstay for the treatment of DKA exists. Overzealous administration, particularly fluid boluses, should be avoided, especially in children and the elderly, because of the risk of cerebral edema.

Follow-up/Prognosis

A small but definite risk of complications in patients with DKA is present. Specifically, infarction and infection carry appreciable risk of mortality. These entities should be considered in the initial evaluation and management of such patients. Occasionally in patients with type 2 diabetes, especially obese African Americans, DKA occurs. Considered to be atypical, the condition is presumably due to severe reversible β-cell dysfunction. The condition is managed with aggressive fluid resuscitation, followed by discontinuation of insulin after hospitalization.

Patient Education/Prevention

Early recognition and treatment of undiagnosed diabetes mellitus and comorbid conditions, as well as administration of drugs that elevate the serum glucose, are essential factors in reducing the incidence of DKA. After an episode of hyperglycemic decompensation, glycemic control is unlikely to return for several weeks after hospitalization. Sick-day management—that is, patient self-directed care during illness that includes increased glucose monitoring, maintenance of adequate hydration and rest, modification of insulin regimen, and a clear understanding of when to contact the physician (ketonuria, blood sugar >300 mg/dL, difficulty breathing, vomiting, or prolonged diarrhea)—should be taught to all diabetic patients and their caretakers, when appropriate. An identification bracelet (e.g., Medic Alert) should be worn at all times. Individuals with recurrent DKA should be managed by a multidisciplinary team.

HYPERGLYCEMIC, HYPEROSMOLAR NONKETOTIC COMA (HHNC)

HHNC is defined as a blood glucose greater than 400–600 mg, impairment of mental status, and an osmolarity of greater than 320 mOsm/kg (18,19). Dehydration is severe without significantly associated ketoacidosis. Although uncommon, HHNC usually occurs in elderly patients with type 2 diabetes. Iatrogenesis, nursing home or family neglect, and poisoning are also recognized precipitants. Careful, aggressive fluid and electrolyte resuscitation combined with vigilance for unsuspected serious illness can minimize the significant mortality of HHNC.

Chief Complaint

Most patients complain of nonspecific symptoms, such as thirst. Mental status may be altered.

Clinical Manifestations

Polyuria, polydipsia, tachycardia, and low-grade fever are fairly characteristic. Neurologic findings range from lateralized findings of aphasia, hemiparesis, hemianopsia, hemisensory defects, and eye deviation to myoclonic jerks, nystagmus, seizures, autonomic dysfunction (hypertension and hyperpnea), Babinski reflexes, and hypo- or hypertonicity. Fewer than 10%–20% of cases are associated with coma. Level of consciousness is best correlated with the serum osmolarity, particularly above levels of 330 mOsm/L, and not with the serum glucose or degree of acidosis. The calculated effective osmolarity is a much better index of serum tonicity than is serum osmolarity.

Although the incidence of HHNC is approximately one-sixth that of DKA, important shared features, as well as distinctive characteristics (Table 5.9), do exist.

T ABLE 5.9.   Clinical comparison

Factor	DKA	HHNC	Both
Age/sex	Young	Old	Female sex
Underlying conditions	Trauma	Acromegaly, Cushing's syndrome, thyrotoxicosis, subdural hematoma, renal failure, hypothermia, pulmonary embolism, surgery	Previously undiagnosed diabetes mellitus, acute infections, pancreatitis, shock and hypovolemia, myocardial infarction, cerebrovascular accident
Comorbid conditions		Hypertension, renal disease, heart failure	Psychiatric illness, alcoholism
Medications		Diuretics, glucocorticoids, parenteral or enteral nutrition, other	Insufficient insulin level

DKA, diabetic ketoacidosis; HHNC, hyperglycemic hyperosmolar nonketotic coma.

Risk Factors

New-onset diabetes mellitus occurs in 17%-25% of HHNC cases (18-21). In 35%-60% of patients, an underlying infection, particularly of the pulmonary or urinary tract, is present. Discontinued insulin accounts for 0%-35% of HHNC cases. Miscellaneous etiologic factors, which account for 10%-15% of HHNC cases, are important causes and are largely iatrogenic. Water loss, medications, such as immunosuppressive drugs, calcium channel blockers, chlorpromazine (Thorazine), diuretics, steroids, beta blockers, diazoxide, phenytoin (Dilantin), loxapine (Loxatane), and cimetidine (Tagamet), enteral or parenteral nutrition, surgery (postcardiac), and increased osmotic loads can cause HHNC. Other causes are pancreatitis, heat stroke, pulmonary embolus, severe burns, myocardial and cerebral infarction, dialysis, and rhabdomyolysis.

Epidemiologic Factors

Females and the elderly are more commonly affected than males and younger adults, although children with type 2 diabetes mellitus have developed HHNC. The incidence of HHNC is about 2.3 per 100,000 person-years, with the most common age range being 55-70 years. The mortality rate is 8%-35%.

Pathophysiology

See Fig. 5.2.

Diagnosis

Altered mental status in conjunction with elevated osmolarity and serum glucose confirms the diagnosis. However, DKA (Table 5.10) and other illnesses that alter the sensorium should be considered (e.g., myocardial and cerebral infarction, sepsis, electrolyte disturbance, etc.).

Referral

All patients with HHNC require hospitalization and management in an intensive care setting. Consultation with an endocrinologist is advisable.

Management

Management of HHNC consists of intravenous (IV) access with a large-bore catheter, aggressive fluid resuscitation (2-3 L of normal saline) with insulin and electrolytes according to the guidelines for DKA, and immediate transportation to the closest ED (20,21). The degree of dehydration in HHNC is greater than that associated with DKA. Heparin, particularly in the elderly, is recommended because of the risk of thromboembolism. In the elderly, inva-

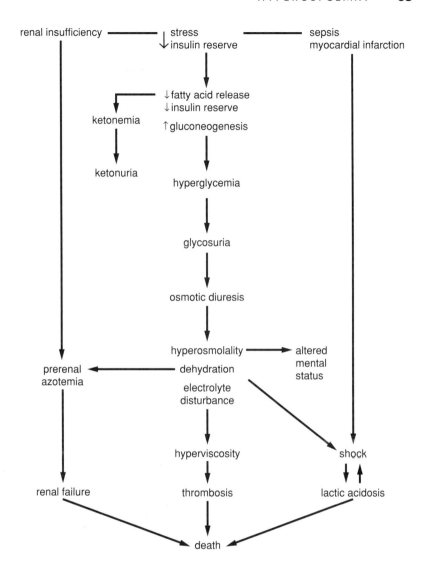

FIGURE 5.2. Pathophysiology of hyperglycemic, hyperosmolar nonketotic coma.

sive monitoring is appropriate in order to avoid fluid overload. Complications are rhabdomyolysis, acute respiratory distress syndrome, shock, thromboembolism, and electrolyte abnormalities. Cerebral edema can develop with overly rapid correction of serum osmolarity, particularly in children. Prognosis depends on levels of BUN, serum sodium, blood glucose, and serum osmolarity.

T ABLE 5.10. Clinical findings in DKA and HHNC

Finding	DKA	HHNC
Patient age	Young (<40)	Middle-aged to elderly (>40)
Type of diabetes diagnosed	Insulin-dependent (type 1)	Non-insulin-dependent (type 2)
Duration of decomposition	Hours to days	Days to weeks
Polyuria, polydipsia	Yes	Yes
Nausea, vomiting	Yes	Yes
Change in mental status	Variable	Yes
Acetone in breath	Yes	No
Kussmaul's respirations	Yes	No
Abdominal pain, tenderness	Yes	No
Tachycardia	Yes	Yes
Glucose	<1000 mg/dL	>1000 mg/dL
Sodium	<140 mEq/L	>140 mEq/L
Potassium	Variable	Often high
Osmolality	mgh/mgh-normal	>330 mOsm/kg
BUN	<60 mg/dL	>60 mg/dL
Bicarbonate	very low (<15)	Normal or slightly decreased (>20)
Muscular sensitivity	+	+++
pH	<7.3	>63
Ketonuria	>3+	<1+
Underlying conditions	Trauma, pulmonary embolism, pancreatitis, stroke, surgery	Acromegaly, Cushing's syndrome, thyrotoxicosis, subdural hematoma, renal failure, dialysis, hypothermia, pulmonary embolism, surgery, heart failure, heat stroke, dehydration, cerebral or myocardial infarction, hypertension
Drugs	Alcohol, glucocorticoids	Diuretics, glucocorticoids, parenteral or enteral nutrition, beta and calcium channel blockers, phenytoin, cimetidine, loxapine, chlorpromazine, immunosuppressive agents

DKA, diabetic ketoacidosis; HHNC, hyperglycemic hyperosmolar nonketotic coma; BUN, blood urea nitrogen.

Follow-up/Prognosis

Electrolyte abnormalities, shock, thromboembolism, ARDS, rhabdomyolysis, and cerebral edema have occurred with HHNC. Overly aggressive fluid resuscitation can lead to ARDS and cerebral edema. Complications are more common in the elderly, who typically have comorbid disease. Pediatric patients should be carefully observed for cerebral edema, a fatal complication with an incidence of 1%–8.5%. After the initial episode of HHNC, patients should be carefully followed with regular visits and repeated education regarding premonitory symptoms because the risk of subsequent episodes is significantly higher.

Patient Education/Prevention

Early recognition and treatment of undiagnosed diabetes mellitus, infection, and decreased water intake in the elderly, particularly the nursing home population, facilitate identification and prevention of HHNC. Drugs that increase the serum glucose in individuals with type 2 diabetes mellitus should be replaced, or appropriate changes in insulin or oral hypoglycemic agents should be made. Sick-day management—that is, patient self-directed care during illness that includes increased glucose monitoring, maintenance of adequate hydration and rest, modification of insulin regimen, a clear understanding of when to contact the physician (ketonuria, blood sugar >300 mg/dL, difficulty breathing, vomiting, or prolonged diarrhea), and the provision of a caretaker, if appropriate—is important. An identification bracelet (e.g., Medic Alert) should be worn at all times.

REFERENCES

12. Lebovitz HE. Diabetic ketoacidosis. *Lancet* 1995;345:767–772.

13. Harper DE, Waldrop RD. Infant diabetic ketoacidosis in the emergency department. *South Med J* 1996;89(7):729–731.

14. Glaser NS, Kuppermann N, Yec CK, et al. Variation in the management of pediatric diabetic ketoacidosis by specialty training. *Arch Pediatr Adolesc Med* 1997;151:1125–1132.

15. Rosenbloom AL, Hanas R. Diabetic ketoacidosis. treatment guidelines. *Clin Pediatr* 1996;35:261–266.

16. Kitabchi AE, Wall BM. Diabetic ketoacidosis. *Med Clin N Am* 1995;79 (1):9–37.

17. Bell DSH, Alele J. Diabetic ketoacidosis. *Postgrad Med* 1997;101(4): 193–204.

18. Lorber D. Nonketotic hypertonicity in diabetes mellitus. *Med Clin N Am* 1995;79(1):39–52.

19. Cruz-Caudillo JC, Sabatini S. Diabetic hyperosmolar syndrome. *Nephron* 1995;69:201–210.

20. Gonzalez-Campoy JM, Robertson RP. Diabetic ketoacidosis and hyperosmolar nonketotic state. *Postgrad Med* 1996;99(6):143–152.

21. Umpierrez GE, Khajavi M, Kitabchi AE. Review: diabetic ketoacidosis and hyperglycemic hyperosmolar nonketotic syndrome. *Am J Med Sci* 1996; 311(5):225–233.

Adrenal Crisis

Unlike adrenal insufficiency, adrenal crisis is an acute, life-threatening emergency that must be suspected and treated on clinical grounds alone. The condition is due primarily to critical cortisone and secondarily to aldosterone insufficiencies and may represent either an exacerbation of long-standing disease (more common) or a *de novo* case. A crisis occurs when the physiologic demand for both hormones exceeds the capacity of the adrenal glands to produce them. Acute insufficiency may occur in patients of any age, from neonates to the elderly, and from a wide range of causes. Though rare, it is a readily treatable condition.

CHIEF COMPLAINTS

1. Altered mental status and unexplained weakness following an office procedure or other major stressor
2. Sudden unexplained shock following a serious infection

CLINICAL MANIFESTATIONS

Patients appear acutely ill or profoundly weak, and may be confused. Check for a background history of corticosteroid use and any recent stressors. Unexplained hypotension (<110 mm Hg), particularly postural hypotension, is present in 80%–90% of patients and may be the sole clue. Circulatory collapse may be profound and may be refractory to large volumes of saline. The pulse is feeble and rapid, and the heart sounds may be soft. Although adrenal crisis commonly elevates body temperature, infection should always be considered. Nausea and vomiting are present in 50%–90% of cases, and anorexia and weight loss are almost universal. Abdominal pain (in 30%–40% of cases) may be severe, suggesting an acute abdomen, replete with distention, rigidity, and rebound tenderness. More than 75% of individuals with primary insufficiency (Addison's disease) present with mucocutaneous hyperpigmentation, particularly in areas of trauma and friction. If the etiology is autoimmune, vitiligo may be observed. Individuals with adrenal hemorrhage more characteristically have abdominal, flank, back, or chest pain. Increased motor activity, which can progress to delirium or seizures, may occur. Typical mental status changes include confusion, lethargy, disorientation, depressed mentation, seizures, and coma.

RISK FACTORS

A number of well-defined precipitating factors can lead to an adrenal crisis. Examples include pyrogens, myocardial and cerebral infarction, alcohol, hypothermia, asthma, trauma, volume loss, anesthesia, surgery, pain, psychotic break, depression, and hypoglycemia.

T ABLE 5.11. Causes of acute primary adrenal insufficiency (22,23)

- Adrenal apoplexy (bilateral infarction or hemorrhage secondary to anticoagulation or idiopathic adrenal vein thrombosis) (23)
- Sepsis (especially from *Meningococcus* or *Pseudomonas* sp.) (Waterhouse-Friderichsen syndrome)
- Hypermetabolic states (diabetes, hyperthyroidism)
- Minor or major procedural interventions (venography)
- Burns
- Convulsions
- Pregnancy

EPIDEMIOLOGIC FACTORS

Chronic primary adrenal insufficiency is idiopathic in 65%–80% of cases and is secondary to tuberculosis in 20% of cases. The remaining causes are rare and include AIDS, certain drugs (hypnotics and general anesthetics), a variety of infective agents and infiltrative disorders (sarcoidosis, neoplasia, amyloidosis), hereditary disorders, and adrenalectomy. Of the idiopathic causes, 70%–75% are autoimmune and are associated with diabetes mellitus, pernicious anemia, thyroiditis, ovarian failure, vitiligo, hypoparathyroidism, malabsorption, and chronic active hepatitis. Table 5.11 lists the causes of acute primary adrenal insufficiency.

Patients are most at risk between day 3 and day 18 of induction of anticoagulation therapy.

The most common cause of adrenal insufficiency is chronic glucocorticoid administration. A general measure of risk is the "rule of twos." The administration of glucocorticoids (cortisone or its equivalent) at a dosage of more than 20 mg daily, orally or parenterally, for a continuous 2 weeks within the past 2 years suggests secondary adrenocortical suppression. Cortisol production in response to stress may be impaired for up to a year after discontinuation. Much rarer causes of secondary adrenal insufficiency include pituitary and hypothalamic diseases and their associated radiation and surgical treatments.

PATHOPHYSIOLOGY

The adrenal gland consists of an outer cortex and inner medulla. The cortex produces life-essential glucocorticoid, mineralocorticoid, and androgenic steroid hormones. The medulla secretes epinephrine and norepinephrine, catecholamines that are largely under neural control. Before clinical manifestations of adrenal failure occur, 90% of the cortex must be involved. In Addison's disease (primary adrenal insufficiency), the gland itself cannot produce cortisol or aldosterone. In secondary adrenal insufficiency, the locus of failure is the hypothalamic–pituitary axis. It is usually characterized by decreased adrenocorticotropic hormone (ACTH) secretion and blunted cortisol production, but aldosterone levels remain normal due to stimulation by hyperkalemia and the renin–angiotensin axis.

The majority of manifestations associated with adrenal insufficiency develop when the physiologic requirement for mineralocorticoid and glucocorticoid hormones exceeds the capacity of the adrenal glands to secrete them. Hypotension is secondary to depressed myocardial contractility from cortisol deficiency and to reduced catecholamine responsiveness and hypovolemia if aldosterone deficiency is also present. The hypotension elevates the BUN and hematocrit. Compensatory ACTH and melanocyte-stimulating hormone secretion produce hyperpigmentation. Depressed gluconeogenesis and increased peripheral glucose use secondary to lipolysis lead to hypoglycemia. Elevated antidiuretic hormone and decreased glomerular filtration rate lower sodium levels. Hyperkalemia results from a depressed glomerular filtration rate, aldosterone deficiency, and acidosis.

DIAGNOSTIC TESTING

Blood should be drawn to measure electrolytes and glucose and to identify the precipitating cause of the crisis. Azotemia secondary to dehydration and acidosis secondary to vascular collapse are usually present in the setting of acute bilateral adrenal hemorrhage. If a background of adrenal insufficiency is present, an electrolyte study, if available, will usually yield a moderately decreased serum sodium level (80% from primary causes, 15% from secondary); but electrolytes may also be normal. Potassium levels are usually normal to slightly increased (60% in primary cases). Rarely, potassium concentration can be markedly increased, causing cardiac arrhythmias or hyperkalemic paralysis. Hypoglycemia is more characteristic of secondary cases (50%), compared with primary (25%), and can be severe. Hypercalcemia is present in 6% of primary cases.

DIAGNOSIS

The diagnosis of acute adrenal insufficiency should include a consideration of possible myxedema (high thyroid-stimulating hormone levels), sepsis (positive blood cultures, source), severe heart failure (peripheral edema, ascites, hepatomegaly, etc.), tamponade (Virchow's triad), severe acidosis (marked decrease in pH), and severe hypocalcemia (severely decreased serum calcium).

REFERRAL

All patients who develop an acute adrenal crisis require hospitalization, usually in an intensive or critical care unit. An endocrinologic consultation should be ordered for management and diagnostic purposes.

MANAGEMENT

Therapeutic measures should be instituted immediately, based on clinical impression, and should not be delayed for confirmatory testing of adrenal function (24). A large-bore IV access line should be established to administer fluids, glucocorticoids, and glucose. Fifty to 100 milliliters of 50% glucose in water should be immediately given for symptomatic hypoglycemia or extremely low serum levels (see hypoglycemia earlier in this chapter).

Correction of dehydration, hypotension, hyponatremia, and hypoglycemia is best accomplished by a rapid infusion of normal saline and 5% glucose in the hospital setting (24). Typically, the extracellular volume deficit in such patients is about 3 L (more with primary causes and less with secondary causes) or approximately 20%. The first liter should be administered over 1 hour, and 2–3 L may be required during the first 8 hours of therapy. Because the functional capacity of the cardiovascular system is reduced with adrenal insufficiency, caution is advised with the rapid administration of saline. A water-soluble glucocorticoid should be administered promptly. Hydrocortisone sodium succinate (Solu-Cortef) or phosphate, 100 mg, should be given as an IV bolus. Intramuscular administration is not sufficient because it is absorbed too slowly to provide adequate cortisol levels to prevent shock. In addition, 100 mg of hydrocortisone should be added to the IV solution. Usually 100–200 mg of hydrocortisone is given every 6 hours during the first 24 hours of therapy; this corrects hyponatremia, hyperkalemia, hypoglycemia, and hypotension. Dexamethasone phosphate, 4 mg every 6–8 hours given intravenously, can also be used because the drug does not factitiously elevate serum cortisol determinations. A mineralocorticoid therapy is not required during initial treatment of adrenal crisis because high doses of corticosteroids provide sufficient mineralocorticoid effect. Empirical stress doses of IV steroids must be given whenever the diagnosis of adrenal crisis is considered and should never be withheld from a symptomatic or unstable patient while awaiting confirmatory lab reports.

If hypotension persists despite adequate volume resuscitation and corticosteroid replacement, additional corticosteroids should be given. Other causes of hypotension should be investigated. Vasopressors may be needed to correct the hypotension, but it is often pressor resistant. Concomitant administration of anticoagulants should prompt consideration of adrenal hemorrhage.

FOLLOW-UP/PROGNOSIS

After initiation of appropriate therapy, the crisis should begin to resolve favorably within a few hours. Since intense treatment or monitoring should continue for 24 to 48 hours, the patient should be referred for immediate hospital admission. Most patients with adrenal crisis do well following prompt recognition and appropriate treatment. Patients who are not treated and those who have adrenal crisis secondary to bilateral adrenal hemorrhage

T ABLE 5.12. Management of chronic adrenal insufficiency

Minor Febrile Illness or Stress
- Increase glucocorticoid dose two- to threefold for illness lasting a few days; do not modify mineralocorticoid.
- If illness persists for more than 3 days, contact physician.

Emergency Treatment of Severe Trauma or Stress
- Inject contents of prefilled dexamethasone syringe (4 mg) intramuscularly.
- Seek medical help as soon as possible.

Hospitalization
- For moderate illness, administer 50 mg hydrocortisone twice daily IV or orally; taper rapidly to maintenance as patient recovers.
- For severe illness, administer 100 mg hydrocortisone every 8 hrs, taper to maintenance by decreasing by half every day.
- For moderately stressful procedures (e.g., endoscopy, arteriography), give a single 100-mg IV dose of hydrocortisone immediately preceding the procedure.
- For major surgery, give 100 mg hydrocortisone IV just before anesthesia induction and continue every 8 hr for first 24 h. Taper rapidly thereafter, decreasing by half per day, to maintenance level.

have high morbidity and mortality rates from hyperkalemia-induced cardiac arrhythmias, hypoglycemia, and circulatory collapse. Patients who are successfully diagnosed and treated require careful follow-up to avert another crisis that may be caused by the development of a comorbid condition or by failure to adhere to the medication regimen.

PATIENT EDUCATION/PREVENTION

Although an increase or supplementation of steroids is not necessary for a relatively short, routine office procedure (e.g., minor surgery, endoscopy, etc.), stress must be minimized in the patient with adrenal insufficiency. A morning appointment is desirable; IV or other sedative and good pain control should be considered to reduce crisis risk. In general, the patient should be instructed to double the usual daily dosage of glucocorticoid during periods of stress, such as infection or metabolic decompensation (diabetes, thyroid disease, immune suppression, etc.), and to notify the family physician. Table 5.12 gives guidelines for corticosteroid use in patients with adrenal insufficiency.

REFERENCES

22. Oelkers W. Adrenal insufficiency. *N Engl J Med* 1996;335(16):1206–12.

23. Rao RH, Vagnucci AH, Amico JA. Bilateral massive adrenal hemorrhage: early recognition and treatment. *Ann Intern Med* 1989;110:227–350.

24. Malchoff CD, Carey RM. Adrenal insufficiency. *Curr Ther Endocrinol Metab* 1997;6:142–147.

CHAPTER 6

....

Neurologic

James E. Nahlik

ALTERED MENTAL STATUS

In the office setting many possible causes of altered mental status or neurologic deficit are found. The differential diagnosis for altered mental status includes conditions that are associated with significant morbidity and mortality. Thus, the care of these patients must be rapid and thorough. The resources required to ensure and maintain cardiopulmonary stabilization and to perform the initial workup include oxygen, nitroglycerin, intravenous (IV) materials, and a well-trained staff.

Chief Complaint

Patients with altered mental status report a wide variety of symptoms, and their concerns are often varied and sometimes vague. In some cases, the patient does not have an accurate memory of recent events. Ideally, a friend or family member will be able to clear up any inconsistencies, such as whether the patient sustained head trauma or experienced emesis. The patient with acute delirium often simply cannot say much about himself or herself. The essential features of delirium include disturbances of consciousness, attention, cognition, and perception. These disturbances develop over a short period of time (usually hours to days) and tend to fluctuate during the course of the day.

Clinical Manifestations

Patients with acute delirium often appear poorly dressed or have poor hygiene. On examination, they are slow to respond to questions and are unable to answer some inquiries. The patient with mild impairment appears normal on cursory examination. The patient with more severe changes sometimes is dyspneic or diaphoretic. Depending on the etiologic factors, the mental status changes can be associated with a number of nonspecific neurologic findings, such as tremor, myoclonus asterixis, and reflex or muscle tone changes. For example, nystagmus and ataxia may accompany delirium caused by medication intoxication; cerebellar signs, myoclonus, and generalized hyperreflexia may be seen with lithium intoxication; cranial nerve palsies may occur with Wernicke's encephalopathy; and asterixis may be observed with renal or hepatic insufficiency.

Risk Factors

Advanced age is the most important risk factor for altered mental status. Other factors include acute trauma, infection (e.g., infection with HIV), and ingestion of substances such as alcohol. Increased age and metabolic or hormonal disorders (e.g., diabetes) may also play a role.

Epidemiologic Factors

The prevalence of delirium in the hospitalized medically ill ranges from 10% to 30%. Among the hospitalized elderly, the delirium prevalence ranges from 10% to 40%. As many as 25% of hospitalized patients with cancer and 30%–40% of hospitalized patients with AIDS have delirium. It is present in as many as 51% of postoperative patients and in up to 80% of patients with a terminal illness who are near death. Patients who have just had surgery, particularly cardiotomy, or hip surgery or transplantation, patients with burns or central nervous system lesions, and those who undergo dialysis are at increased risk for delirium. Conditions that are most amenable to quality improvement include heart disease, undernutrition, dementia, and depression. These are all common diagnoses in the office practice, and it behooves the physician to be ready for their presentation in acute distress.

Pathophysiology

The patient's level of consciousness can be described along a continuum from alert to drowsy to stuporous to comatose. Literally hundreds of chemical agents and disease entities exist that can alter mental status. Whereas the patient with more gradual changes may well have dementia, acute delirium should be considered in the patient with acute changes.

Diagnosis

On examination, the vital signs, including temperature, blood pressure, respiratory rate, pulse, height, and weight, should be thoroughly documented. Abnormalities in these measurements may steer the clinician to the affected organ system. Proper evaluation and initial management include evaluation of metabolic factors and assessment for toxic ingestion, as well as a thorough neurologic assessment. The patient must also be given the Mini-Mental State Examination (Table 6.1), a useful verbal assessment of the patient's degree of functionality. When acute delirium is suspected, evidence from the history, physical examination, or laboratory tests usually suggests a general medical cause, substance intoxication or withdrawal, medication use, toxin exposure, or a combination of these. A typical issue in the differential diagnosis of mental status changes is distinguishing (a) dementia from delirium and (b) delirium alone from delirium that is superimposed on preexisting dementia. Cognitive disturbances, such as memory impairment, are common to both delirium and dementia; however, the patient with dementia usually is alert

T ABLE 6.1. Mini-Mental State Examination

Task	Instructions	Scoring	Total points
Date orientation	"Tell me the date." Ask for omitted items.	One point each for year, season, date, day of week, and month	5
Place orientation	"Where are you?" Ask for omitted items.	One point each for state, county, town, building, and floor or room	5
Register 3 objects	Name three objects slowly and clearly. Ask the patient to repeat them.	One point for each item correctly repeated	3
Serial sevens	Ask the patient to count backward from 100 by 7. Stop after five answers. (Or ask patient to spell "world" backward.)	One point for each correct answer (or letter)	5
Recall 3 objects	Ask the patient to recall the objects mentioned above.	One point for each item correctly remembered	3
Naming	Point to your watch and ask the patient, "What is this?" Repeat with a pencil.	One point for each correct answer	2
Repeating a phrase	Ask the patient to say "no ifs, ands, or buts."	One point if successful on first try	1
Verbal commands	Give the patient a plain piece of paper and say, "Take this paper in your right hand, fold it in half, and put it on the floor."	One point for each correct action	3
Written commands	Show the patient a piece of paper with "Close Your Eyes" printed on it.	One point if the patient's eyes close	1
Writing	Ask the patient to write a sentence.	One point if sentence has a subject, a verb, and makes sense	1
Drawing	Ask the patient to copy a pair of intersecting pentagons onto a piece of paper.	One point if the figure has 10 corners and 2 intersecting lines	1
Scoring	Total possible is 30; a score of 24 or above is considered normal.		

Adapted from Folstein MF, Folstein SE, McHugh PR. Mini-mental state: a practical method for grading the cognitive state of patients for the clinician. *J Psych Res* 1975;12:189–198.

and does not have the disturbance of consciousness or arousal that is characteristic of delirium. Psychiatric illness, such as bipolar disorder or schizophrenia, must also be considered.

Management

The initial evaluation should begin with an assessment of airway, breathing, and circulatory status (the "ABCs"). Because vitamin B deficiency, hypoglycemia, or opiate toxicity may be the cause of altered mental status, 100 mg of thiamine (Thiamilate), 25-50 g of 50% glucose, or 1 to 2 mg (up to 10 mg) of naloxone (Narcan) should be given empirically. Before glucose is given, a rapid serum glucose level should be established using a fingerstick sample. Also, if thiamine is to be administered, this should be done before the glucose is given so as not to precipitate or exacerbate Wernicke's encephalopathy.

As the patient is being stabilized, attention is directed to the differential diagnosis. Possibilities include drug toxicity and overdose, metabolic derangements, head injury, cerebrovascular accidents, and infections of the central nervous system. The degree of impairment can be established by discussing the patient's previous functionality with other persons close to the patient. If these conversations confirm that the patient is usually mentally intact, then changes are classified as acute and should be appropriately documented.

Referral

Most patients with altered mental status are referred for hospitalization. Some patients benefit from seeing a neurologist, psychiatrist, or other mental health professional.

Follow-up/Prognosis

The prognosis in these patients is completely dependent on finding a cause and adequately addressing that cause. Although the majority of patients recover fully, patients with delirium may progress to stupor, coma, seizures, or death, particularly if untreated. Full recovery is less likely in the elderly, with estimated rates of full recovery by the time of discharge varying from 4% to 40%. Persistent cognitive deficits are also common in elderly patients recovering from delirium, although such deficits may be due to preexisting dementia that was not fully appreciated. Delirium in the medically ill is associated with significant morbidity. Medically ill patients, particularly the elderly, have a significantly increased risk of developing complications, such as pneumonia and decubitus ulcers, resulting in longer hospital stays. In postoperative patients, delirium is a harbinger of limited recovery and poor long-term outcome. Patients who develop delirium, particularly after orthopedic surgery, are at increased risk for postoperative complications, longer postoperative recuperation periods, longer hospital stays, and long-term disability.

Patient Education/Prevention

The patient needs education about the risk for recurrence of his or her particular altered mental state. The family or a support person must be educated and supported through this time of acute stress.

SEIZURES

If a patient has a seizure in the office, the staff should be ready to respond at once. The patient must be kept safe from self-harm with tonic movements. After a first seizure, evaluation should focus on excluding an underlying neurologic or medical condition, assessing the relative risk of seizure recurrence, and determining whether treatment is indicated. Successful management of patients with recurrent seizures begins with the establishment of an accurate diagnosis, followed by treatment with an appropriate medication.

Chief Complaint

The patient with seizures may describe the loss of control of bodily functions, such as the ability to speak or control movements of the extremities. Often, an observing family member or friend describes these events; and the patient is distressed by the abrupt change in his or her condition. If an acute seizure occurs in the office, the patient may be unable to speak. The staff assistant should be asked to describe the episode to the physician.

Clinical Manifestations

The acute neurologic examination may show focal abnormalities, such as increased reflexes or flaccid muscles; or it may be normal. The patient who has just had an acute seizure may display evidence of incontinence or, more often, the somnolence of the postictal state. Some patients show signs of tongue biting and may describe provoking factors.

Risk Factors

Patients who are at risk for seizures are those with prior seizures, head trauma, alcohol abuse, or a family history of seizures. The most common presentation is a patient who has had prior seizures and who is experiencing subtherapeutic control with current medications. Although seizures in this type of patient most often result from noncompliance, they can also be caused by drug–drug interactions or metabolic changes.

Epidemiologic Factors

Epileptic seizures are a common and important medical problem, with about 1 in 11 persons experiencing at least one seizure at some point. Epilepsy (the tendency to experience recurrent, unprovoked seizures) occurs with a prevalence of about 0.5% and a cumulative lifetime incidence of 3%. The management of patients with epilepsy is often challenging, as evidenced by a recent report that more than half of all patients with epilepsy continue to experience at least occasional seizures despite treatment with antiepileptic medications. New clinical advances offer considerable hope for these patients.

Pathophysiology

A seizure is an outpouring of uncoordinated electrical impulses in the brain. Electrical dysfunction in the brain is the common element in all seizures. Nerve cells in the brain communicate by way of electrical signals; but when this activity becomes disorganized, the exchange between nerve cells is thrown into chaos, and a seizure results.

Many seizures occur in the three stages described below.

- *Aura.* A warning period during which a person experiences symptoms (such as a feeling of fear or impending doom or an unpleasant odor or taste) that signal an approaching attack.
- *Ictus.* The stage in which the most dramatic electrical disorganization occurs. Symptoms vary widely and can include prolonged staring spells, odd behaviors, loss of consciousness, and convulsions.
- *Postictus.* The minutes or hours of abnormal consciousness after the seizure. A person may feel sleepy or confused. Parts of the body may feel weak or even paralyzed, although this is temporary. During the postictal period, the brain is recovering from the seizure and is returning to normal function.

The four broad categories of epilepsy syndromes are:

- Idiopathic generalized
- Symptomatic generalized
- Idiopathic localization-related
- Symptomatic localization-related

In the acute phase, the physician often cannot distinguish between these syndromes. The syndrome of greatest concern is prolonged generalized convulsions, or convulsive status epilepticus. This syndrome may be life-threatening and requires prompt medical attention. With detailed collection of information over time, the pathophysiologic factors, which exert substantial influence in terms of treatment and choice of medications, can be determined.

Diagnosis

Diagnosis of the first seizure is based predominantly on the patient's medical history. Many paroxysmal events may be confused with epileptic seizures, including syncope (see next section), movement disorders (such as tics or tardive dyskinesia), parasomnias (narcolepsy), and psychogenic seizures. These seizure-like events are different in that they affect only distinct parts of the body, such as tics on the face. Diagnostic studies must be tailored to the individual patient. In the patient with a prior history of seizures, serum levels of the current anticonvulsant and a drug screen should be obtained. The patient will be stabilized in the office, and after hospital admission the workup can be detailed. Basic laboratory evaluation focuses on detecting systemic disturbances that are potentially associated with seizures and includes a complete blood count and measurements of electrolytes, calcium, prothrombin time (PT), partial thromboplastin time (PTT), magnesium, phosphorus, blood urea nitrogen, creatinine, glucose, and possibly serum levels of antiseizure medications. If the patient has a history of alcohol or drug use, consider obtaining a toxicology screen and evaluating hepatic function with synthetic and enzyme studies. Lumbar puncture is essential in febrile patients in whom meningitis or encephalitis is suspected, as well as in immunocompromised patients (occult meningitis is a common finding in this group). Computed tomography (CT) of the brain may show an acute cause. Electroencephalography is often helpful in the evaluation of patients presenting with a seizure. The electroencephalogram (EEG) should be obtained within 24 hours of the event, if possible. If it is negative, then it can be followed up with an EEG taken in the sleep-deprived state. The utility of the EEG includes visualization of epileptiform activity, which strengthens the diagnosis; identification of focal electrocerebral abnormalities, which suggests a focal structural brain lesion; and documentation of specific epileptiform patterns associated with particular epilepsy syndromes (e.g., generalized spike-and-wave discharges associated with a generalized epilepsy or focal discharges associated with a localization-related epilepsy).

Management

Protecting patients from self-inflicted harm is key in the office management of acute seizure. A bite stick made of a tongue depressor wrapped in tape can be kept on hand and should be inserted over the tongue to prevent lacerations. Vital signs should be monitored closely. Padding may be provided to reduce traumatic injury. Supplemental oxygen should be provided by mask. A large-bore IV line should be placed. The patient can be given IV lorazepam (Ativan), 2–4 mg, to halt the seizure. When the seizure stops, the patient must be monitored for respiratory depression and, if necessary, should be intubated.

The goal of long-term therapy is to control seizures completely without producing unacceptable side effects. The most important step is to select an antiepileptic drug that is appropriate for the patient's particular type of epilepsy. Diagnosis of a specific epilepsy syndrome is based on the history of the patient's seizure types, neurologic status, and electroencephalographic findings. Treatment of seizures is beyond the scope of this discussion.

Referral

After an acute seizure, the patient usually requires hospitalization for evaluation. One exception may be a child with acute febrile seizures. Patients who do not achieve complete seizure control should be referred to an epilepsy specialist because new medications and surgical treatments offer patients unprecedented options in seizure control.

Follow-up/Prognosis

Although the evaluation and treatment of patients with seizures or epilepsy are often challenging, modern therapy provides many patients with complete seizure control. In addition to considering the probability of recurrence, the physician must also consider the potential psychological, social, and vocational consequences of recurrent seizures. Because children are not as likely to experience severe social or vocational repercussions from a single recurrence, they are rarely treated for a first seizure. However, some adults feel that the consequences of even a single recurrent seizure would dramatically affect their lives, and they may choose to take medication to decrease the chance of a recurrence whether they are at high risk for recurrence or not. Patients who do so should be seen in the office within a month after starting a new anticonvulsant. Such patients often require serum studies to monitor the level of medication and to make dosage adjustments so as to achieve a therapeutic level.

Patient Education/Prevention

Education of the patient with new seizures must begin soon after occurrence of the first seizure. The patient and his or her family will have numerous concerns and questions about the future. Local epilepsy foundations can provide support and education. Proper education about the syndrome can be of great help in encouraging the patient to take his or her medication correctly.

SYNCOPE

Syncope, defined as a sudden and transient loss of consciousness, may result from vasovagal reaction, coronary artery disease, carotid lesions, or metabolic imbalances. Most causes of syncope produce a dramatic fall in blood pressure, which leads to fainting. The patient who faints in the physician's office should be treated for shock and requires a thorough neurologic examination.

Chief Complaint

Patients generally describe syncopal episodes using terms such as "passing out," "blackout," "flipping out," or "sleep attacks."

The description of the syncopal event, including duration of unconsciousness, rapidity of recovery, seizure activity, changes in skin color, and presence of diaphoresis, should be obtained from those who witnessed the event

Clinical Manifestations

Studies in which volunteers were videotaped during induced syncopal events illustrate the common occurrence of repetitive clonic, myoclonic, or dystonic movements associated with fainting. However, these movements rarely persist beyond 5–10 seconds and do not exhibit the organized progression from tonic to clonic phase that is characteristic of a convulsive seizure. Thus, a detailed history of the motor activity, together with the usual questions regarding premonitory symptoms, provoking factors, tongue biting, incontinence, and the postictal state, can often help distinguish between syncope and seizures. Unlike the patient who has seizures, the patient with syncope does not usually display a postictal drowsiness, tongue biting, or incontinence. The patient with true syncope may report dizziness, palpitations, and chest pain. Occasionally, headache is associated with syncope.

Risk Factors

True syncope can sometimes be traced to underlying coronary artery disease, carotid lesions, or metabolic imbalances. Although the causes of syncope may be heterogeneous, the timing, descriptions, and clinical course suggest that many reported cases are caused by vasovagal reaction. Vasovagal fainting may occur in association with the administration of vaccines; many patients who experience such fainting do so within 15 minutes of vaccination.

Epidemiologic Factors

Nearly half of all Americans will experience at least one episode of syncope during their lifetime. Syncope occurs in people of all ages. More than 100,000 patients per year present to a physician reporting repeated episodes of syncope. Syncope accounts for 3% of all visits to the emergency department and 1% of hospital admissions. In patients in whom a cause was established, 30% were attributed to vasovagal factors; 30% were attributed to cardiac factors; 10% were orthostatic; 10% were induced by drugs; and 8% were situational.

Pathophysiology

Syncope results from inadequate delivery of oxygen or metabolic substrate to the brain or from disorganized electrical activity in the brain. An accumulation of these conditions may diminish cerebral oxygen delivery, pushing it dangerously close to the threshold needed to maintain consciousness. Any stress that further reduces cerebral blood flow or blood oxygen content may precipitate syncope. Syncope, or near-syncope, is usually secondary to a disorder of the cardiovascular system that causes systemic hypotension and, thus, collapse. Vasovagal reaction is a common syndrome that is caused by hyperstimulation of the sympathetic nervous system in response to pain, fear, or emotional distress. The hyperstimulation is followed by a sudden onset of hypotension, which often results in syncope. Syncopal seizures may also develop secondary to transient cerebral anoxia.

Diagnosis

The diagnosis of syncope is clinical and can be established through a complete history of the event and the recovery period. Recovery from syncope is usually rapid; however, when a syncopal event follows a seizure, recovery tends to be slow. To rule out orthostatic hypotension, check blood pressure and heart rate with the patient in the supine position after he or she has rested for 5 minutes. If possible, have the patient stand for 1 minute and 3 minutes; and check the blood pressure and heart rate after each interval. A small increase or no increase in heart rate upon standing may suggest baroreflex impairment. An exaggerated increase in heart rate upon standing may indicate volume depletion.

The carotid arteries should be auscultated for bruits to rule out conditions that contraindicate carotid sinus massage. The heart should be auscultated for murmurs of aortic stenosis, mitral regurgitation, or hypertrophic cardiomyopathy, all of which are common in elderly patients. Mitral regurgitation is marked by a holosystolic murmur at the apex, but such a murmur may also occur in elderly patients who have aortic stenosis or hypertrophic cardiomyopathy. An accentuation of the systolic murmur while the patient performs Valsalva's maneuver helps distinguish hypertrophic cardiomyopathy from aortic stenosis or mitral regurgitation. Neurologic examination to search for focal abnormalities that may indicate cerebrovascular disease or space-occupying lesions is essential.

Specialized studies are generally undertaken only if they are indicated by findings in the history and physical examination. A 12-lead electrocardiogram (ECG) is a valuable tool that may provide a diagnosis of ischemia, arrhythmia, or conduction abnormality in up to 10% of patients. Ideally, patients can be kept on the monitor to identify arrhythmias. A Holter monitor may be a consideration for follow-up in selected patients. Patients with abnormalities such as a carotid bruit must be scheduled for a carotid Doppler scan. In some patients with cardiac murmurs, valuable information can be gained from a transesophageal echocardiogram. The serum studies of value include hematocrit and glucose levels. Serum creatinine kinase may be drawn to assess the degree of muscle trauma and to determine whether IV fluids are indicated. If the patient is taking an antiarrhythmic, an anticonvulsant, a bronchodilator, or lithium, the drug concentration should be measured to determine whether it is subtherapeutic, therapeutic, or toxic. If the concentration is subtherapeutic, the syncopal episode may be the result of inadequate treatment of a known predisposing condition, such as seizure disorder.

Management

The patient who faints in the office should be treated for shock. The patient's legs should be elevated, and a blanket, sheet, or gown should be placed over him or her. Smelling salts (ammonia inhalant, 0.3 mL) can be used as a respiratory stimulant. Vital signs must be monitored. Oxygen by mask can be lifesaving. An ECG or monitor strip taken during the episode can provide valuable diagnostic information. At this time the clinician should perform a thorough neurologic exam. If vital signs deteriorate, full resuscitation protocol and cardiopulmonary resuscitation may be necessary.

Referral

Patients older than 60 years of age and those with heart disease should be admitted to the hospital. Also, patients with abnormalities noted in neurologic or cardiac studies—especially those with an abnormal ECG—should be admitted. No benefit to admission for high-risk patients has been demonstrated, but monitoring and testing may be expedited.

Follow-up/Prognosis

Younger patients without heart disease who have had a single episode of syncope are at no greater risk of sudden death than are their age-matched cohorts. They may be reassured and referred for outpatient follow-up but should be cautioned that a subsequent syncopal episode should prompt a follow-up visit to a physician or to the emergency department. Some patients should be taught to avoid common precipitants of syncope, such as rising from bed too quickly, especially in the middle of the night. Patients with orthostatic hypotension should sit on the edge of the bed and flex their feet before standing. Those with postprandial hypotension may benefit from eating small, frequent meals and lying down after each meal. Walking after a meal may prevent postprandial hypotension, but this approach should be undertaken only with supervision. Elderly patients should avoid straining during defecation by using stool softeners and altering their diet.

Patient Education/Prevention

The patient may need education about fluid requirements. Other patients, who faint as a result of mental stress, may benefit from counseling or relaxation techniques.

Preventing syncope and related injuries following immunizations is feasible. Some episodes may be prevented if health care providers recognize presyncopal signs and symptoms, such as pallor, perspiration, trembling, bradycardia, and hypotension. Patients with these signs and symptoms may need to sit or lie down for 10–15 minutes both before and immediately after immunizations are given. Physicians may want to consider instituting a policy of watching patients for a brief time after they have received an immunization. A cardinal rule is that no shots should be given while a patient is standing up.

STROKE/TRANSIENT ISCHEMIC ATTACK

Stroke is the third leading cause of death after coronary artery disease and cancer, and it continues to have a devastating impact on public health in the United States. In the physician's office, the patient is more likely to describe episodes that may be transient ischemic attacks (TIAs).

Chief Complaint

Typically, the patient who has had a stroke will describe changes of sudden onset in sensation or movement. The patient may describe vague symptoms of a "funny" feeling in the extremities or a sensation of not being able to be dexterous in maneuvers previously carried out with ease. In the office setting, patients are more likely to describe symptoms of a TIA. To qualify as a TIA, the duration of symptoms must be less than 24 hours. These symptoms must be taken very seriously and must be evaluated before they progress to the full stroke.

Clinical Manifestations

Vital signs may be normal in a typical stroke patient. Patients may show skin signs of emboli (Janeway lesions, Osler nodes). Papilledema may be present, as may preretinal hemorrhage. Focal paralysis or abnormal reflexes can be most informative in making the diagnosis. Some patients will demonstrate weakness, altered vision, or motor deficits.

Risk Factors

Hypertension is a powerful predictor of both ischemic and hemorrhagic stroke. Smoking is linked to both ischemic and hemorrhagic stroke. Diabetes is associated with stroke independent of other common comorbidities, such as hypertension, obesity, and hyperlipidemia. Elevated cholesterol has a direct association with ischemic stroke and an inverse relationship with hemorrhagic stroke. Atrial fibrillation and recent myocardial infarction are the most important risk factors in cardiogenic embolism.

Epidemiologic Factors

Eighty percent of strokes are ischemic, including those of thrombotic and embolic etiology. The other 20% are hemorrhagic and include intracerebral and subarachnoid strokes. At least 700,000 new stroke cases appear every year. Although the incidence of ischemic stroke has declined over the last 20 years, the mean age of the population has risen and has resulted in a continual increase in the absolute number of strokes. Recent projections indicate that, by the year 2050, more than 1 million strokes will occur each year in the United States.

Pathophysiology

Neurons are very sensitive to changes in cerebral blood flow. Brain cells die within a few minutes of complete cessation of blood flow. The flow of blood can be blocked by the following:

- Large-vessel thrombosis with low flow.
- Artery-to-artery or cardiogenic embolism or embolism of unknown source.
- Small intracerebral vessel occlusion.

TIAs arise from the same mechanisms as ischemic strokes and are warning signals that a stroke is more likely. These are reversible episodes where the occlusion was reversed in time for the brain to achieve recovery.

Lesions of the carotid circulation produce aphasia, dysarthria, ipsilateral monocular visual loss, contralateral hemiparesis, homonymous hemianopsia, or hemisensory loss. Ischemia in the vertebral-basilar circulation produces unilateral or bilateral weakness, sensory loss, diplopia, ataxia, nystagmus, dysarthria, hoarseness, dysphagia, hearing loss, and vertigo.

Diagnosis

The diagnosis of stroke is based initially on history and on physical examination findings. These findings can vary widely based on the area of the brain affected. The physical examination findings may change as the stroke evolves; documentation of this is important in the office setting. The patient who is thought to be describing a TIA may be admitted; but more often, he or she is scheduled to have carotid Doppler studies. The abrupt onset of a focal deficit without a change in the level of consciousness is characteristic of ischemia and infarction, but this phenomenon may also occur with intracranial hemorrhage, tumor, or migraine. If the diagnosis of acute stroke is secured, then the patient should be closely monitored and should be transferred to the hospital.

CT or magnetic resonance imaging (MRI) of the head is necessary to clarify the structural abnormalities responsible for the patient's symptoms and to guide therapeutic decisions. MRI is more useful for visualizing an ischemic infarction, which may not be seen on CT within the first 36 hours. Intracerebral hemorrhage is revealed by either study.

Management

Controlling blood pressure (while avoiding hypotension), ensuring adequate oxygenation, administering IV glucose, taking precautions against dysphagia/aspiration, considering prophylaxis for venous thrombosis if the patient is unable to walk, suppressing fever if present, and assessing stroke mechanism (e.g., atrial fibrillation, hypertension) are important. Consider thrombolytic and aspirin therapy if the stroke is ischemic and if no contraindications are found. After hospitalization and diagnosis are secure, the patient who has had a noncardioembolic stroke is treated with subcutaneous heparin to prevent deep venous thrombosis. These patients may benefit from IV heparin only if they have a carotid plaque rupture or if the stroke continues to progress (after CT has ruled out hemorrhage). IV heparin may also be used in the patient with vertebrobasilar (posterior) or crescendo TIA. In strokes that are found to have a cardioembolic cause, IV heparin and long-term warfarin (Coumadin) are clearly beneficial over aspirin. The exception to this guideline is strokes caused by rheumatic atrial fibrillation, which are treated with surgery. Clopidogrel (Plavix) should be considered in patients with acetylsalicylic acid (ASA) intolerance, in those who are at high risk for recurrence, and in female patients, who have been shown to be less responsive to ASA.

Referral

The patient who has had a stroke will always need to be admitted to the hospital. The patient who has had a TIA may be admitted, but he or she also can be assessed as an outpatient. Admission is required if symptoms compromise the patient's ability to perform the activities of daily living. A consultation with a neurologist is usually indicated, as he or she can provide guidance on the most efficient course of evaluation and testing.

Follow-up/Prognosis

During the first days of an ischemic stroke, neither progression nor outcome can be predicted. About 20% of patients die in the hospital; the mortality rate increases with age. The extent of neurologic recovery depends on the patient's age and general state of health and on the site and size of the infarct. Impaired consciousness, mental deterioration, aphasia, or severe brain-stem signs suggest a poor prognosis. Complete recovery is uncommon; but the sooner improvement begins, the better the prognosis is. About 50% of patients with moderate or severe hemiplegia, and most patients with milder deficits, recover functionally by the time of discharge and have a clear sensorium, can eventually meet their own basic needs, and can walk adequately, although use of an affected limb may be limited. Any deficit remaining after 6 months is likely to be permanent, although some patients continue to improve slowly. Cerebral infarction recurs relatively often, and each recurrence is likely to add to the neurologic disability. Of stroke survivors, 70% have a decrease in their vocational level, and 16% are institutionalized.

Patient Education/Prevention

Extensive education of the patient and the family is necessary after a stroke or TIA. The medical team must help the patient understand the permanent nature of the damage caused by stroke, and patients must be involved in decisionmaking regarding future therapies and lifesaving and life-sustaining interventions. Detection and treatment of hypertension and hypercholesterolemia, as well as cessation of smoking, are important elements of stroke prevention education. Many patients with significant hypertension do not see a physician or do not adhere to therapy. With continued efforts by individual physicians and their staffs, this important risk factor can be detected and treated.

BRAIN BLEEDS

The intracranial hemorrhage is typically a cataclysmic event that is heralded by severe headache, meningeal signs, and neurologic dysfunction. Approximately half of patients with aneurysmal rupture experience "sentinel headaches" days to weeks before a major hemorrhage.

Chief Complaint

Patients may present with only a headache, or they may have varying degrees of neurologic deficits or changes in consciousness. Diagnosis at this stage may permit treatment before a devastating neurologic event occurs.

Clinical Manifestations

Severe unrelenting headaches, sometimes accompanied by nausea and vomiting, characterize the sentinel headaches associated with intracranial hemorrhage. Assessment of vital signs may show elevated blood pressure, and the funduscopic exam may show acute bleeds.

Risk Factors

The main risk factors for brain bleeds are hypertension, family history, head trauma, brain tumors, hypercoagulable states, and use of drugs, such as cocaine or amphetamines. Overall, head trauma is the most common cause of subarachnoid hemorrhage. Spontaneous (primary) subarachnoid hemorrhage usually results from a ruptured congenital intracranial aneurysm. Less commonly, it is caused by a mycotic or arteriosclerotic aneurysm, arteriovenous malformation, or hemorrhagic disease. Aneurysmal hemorrhage may occur at any age, but it is most common in those between 40 to 65 years of age.

Epidemiologic Factors

A subarachnoid hemorrhage occurs in about 1 in 10,000 persons per year in the United States. The hemorrhage is fatal in about 50% of cases.

Pathophysiology

Spontaneous subarachnoid hemorrhage is usually the result of the rupture of an intracranial saccular aneurysm or arteriovenous malformation. The mixture of escaping blood and cerebrospinal fluid irritates the meninges and increases intracranial pressure, producing headache, vomiting, dizziness, and alterations in pulse and respiratory rates. Seizures occasionally occur. The temperature may be elevated during the first 5–10 days; the patient often continues to have headaches and confusion.

Diagnosis

In the office, the patient complains of severe headache. On examination, he or she may be found to have a neurologic deficit. If a change in mental status occurs, emergency evaluation is required. Subarachnoid hemorrhage that is suspected on clinical grounds should be confirmed by CT evaluation. Any new-onset headache or changes in a headache's characteristics must be investigated to exclude aneurysmal subarachnoid hemorrhage and an enlarging aneurysm. A few aneurysms produce symptoms because they press on adjacent structures. Ocular palsies, diplopia, squint, and facial pain indicate pressure on the third, fourth, fifth, or sixth cranial nerve. Visual loss and a bitemporal field defect indicate pressure on the optic chiasm.

Management

Initial treatment of patients with spontaneous subarachnoid hemorrhage includes resuscitation and/or stabilization. The blood pressure should be closely monitored and should be aggressively lowered when necessary. If edema is present, give IV furosemide (Lasix). Once the acute effects of the hemorrhage are managed, arrange prompt referral for neurosurgical treatment.

Referral

If acute bleeding is suspected, the patient should receive oxygen and IV fluids and should be admitted to the hospital at once. At the hospital, urgent consultation with a neurosurgeon is indicated.

Follow-up/Prognosis

Patients with spontaneous subarachnoid hemorrhage have a good prognosis if the correct diagnosis is made early. They should be hospitalized and thereafter should be followed on a frequent basis for several years.

Patient Education

Patient education about subarachnoid hemorrhage includes informing the public that despite the fact that headaches are common and often harmless, an unrelenting headache can signal a serious problem. When an aneurysm ruptures, the headache is usually acute and severe. Any new, severe headache should prompt a visit to the patient's physician or, if he or she is unavailable, to the emergency department.

REFERENCES

1. Miller DK, Coe RM, Morley JE, Romeis JC. *Total quality management in geriatric care.* New York: Springer Publishing, 1995.

2. Folstein MF, Folstein SE, McHugh PR. Mini-Mental State Exam: a practical method for grading the cognitive state of patients for the clinician. *J Psychiatr Res* 1975;12:189-198.

3. Ferrera PC, Chan L. Initial management of the patient with altered mental status. *Am Fam Physician* 1997;55:177-180.

4. Devinsky O. Seizure disorders. *CIBA Clin Symp* 1994;46(1).

5. Linzer M, Yang EH, Estes M. Diagnosing syncope. *Ann Intern Med* 1997; 126:989-996.

6. Braun MM, Patriarca PA, Ellenberg SS. Syncope after immunization. *Arch Pediatr Adolesc Med* 1997;151:255-259.

7. Benavente O, Hart RG. Stroke, Part II. Management of acute ischemic stroke. *Am Fam Physician* 1999;59:10:2828-2834.

8. CAPRIE Steering Committee. A randomised, blinded trial of clopidrogrel versus aspirin in patients at risk of ischemic events (CAPRIE). *Lancet* 1996;348:1329-1339.

9. Beers MH, Berkow R, eds. *Merck manual of diagnosis and therapy*, 17th ed. Whitehouse Station, NJ: Merck and Company, 1999.

CHAPTER 7

....

Surgical

Lloyd A. Darlow and Richard B. Birrer

Patients present to the family physician's office with a full range of medical and surgical conditions, some of which require urgent intervention. Although the family physician infrequently is called on to perform surgical procedures, he or she still has a vital role to play before and, in some cases, after a surgical consult has been obtained.

LACERATIONS

Despite the fact that numerous lacerations occur yearly in the United States, most of them heal without sequelae regardless of how they are managed. However, sometimes wound infections, unsightly and troublesome scars, prolonged convalescence, and, rarely, mortality may result from mismanagement. The goals of laceration management are simple: the achievement of cosmetically and functionally acceptable scars and the avoidance of infection. Establishment of a well-approximated skin closure, debridement of devitalized tissue, reduction of tissue contamination, and restoration of perfusion to poorly perfused wounds optimize outcome.

Epidemiologic Factors

In 1998 approximately 23 million lacerations were treated either in emergency departments or in private physicians' offices on an emergency or urgency basis. One-third of lacerations occur in young adults (19–35 years of age). The majority of patients are male. Fifty percent of cases involve either the head or neck, and 35% involve an upper extremity, usually the fingers or hands. The wound infection rate is relatively low (<5%). The most common mechanism of injury is the application of a blunt force, although sharp instruments, such as glass and wooden objects, also produce lacerations. Lacerations resulting from mammalian bites are relatively rare.

Risk Factors for Wound Infection

Risk factors for wound infection include chronic renal failure, advanced age, corticosteroid use, diabetes mellitus, obesity, and malnutrition. Chemotherapeutic and immunosuppressive agents may delay wound healing by affecting the synthesis of new-wound matrix and by modifying the inflammatory process.

Evaluation

A detailed allergy history is essential because antibiotics and anesthetic agents may be required. Tetanus immunization status must be verified (Table 7.1). The mechanism of injury should be sought, and special attention should be paid to the presence of an undiagnosed foreign body (the fifth leading cause of litigation against emergency physicians). The physician should ask whether the injury is due to crush forces because such injuries have a greater risk of tissue necrosis and more susceptibility to infection.

Examination of the wound should begin with a neurovascular assessment that includes pulses and sensorimotor function distal to the laceration. Sterile gloves, mandated by universal precautions, should be used for the evaluation and repair of routine lacerations, although few studies clearly demonstrate benefits associated with their use.

Anesthesia

Anesthesia of the wound is necessary for adequate evaluation and management. The two major classes of local anesthetics are esters and amides. Little true cross-reactivity is found between them. However, the allergy to lidocaine (Xylocaine) is usually due to the methylparaben preservative used in multidose vials. This methylparaben has a molecular structure similar to that of a degradation product of the ester agents. Thus, substitution of an amide for an ester may be problematic. An alternative is to use single-dose cardiac lidocaine, which does not contain a preservative. The two most commonly used agents are lidocaine and mepivacaine (Carbocaine). The onset of the latter is delayed, but its longer duration of action offers a significant advantage over lidocaine, particularly when prolonged pain is anticipated. Epinephrine anesthetic combinations are contraindicated in the digits and in extremities, such as the nose, ear lobes, and penis.

Buffering of the local anesthetic with sodium bicarbonate in a ratio of 1:10 increases the ratio of uncharged to charged molecules, resulting in a

T ABLE 7.1. Tetanus immunization

History	Clean minor wounds		All other wounds	
	Td	TIG	Td	TIG
≥3 Doses				
Last dose within 5 yr	No	No	No	No
Last dose 5 to 10 yr	No	No	Yes	No
Last dose >10 yr	Yes	No	Yes	No
Uncertain or <3 doses	Yes	No	Yes	Yes

Td, Tetanus-diphtheria toxoid; TIG, tetanus immune globulin.

more rapid and less painful onset of anesthesia. The solution has a shelf life of at least one week. No increase in wound infection rates occurs. Warming of the solution is as effective as buffering. The pain of infiltration can be minimized by the use of a small-bore needle (27- to 30-gauge), by injecting the solution slowly into the subcutaneous (rather than the intradermal) region, and by entering the wounded edges of the laceration instead of the intact surrounding skin. Application of a topical anesthetic before injection, such as 2% topical lidocaine or 1% tetracaine (Pontocaine), attenuates the pain of infiltration. The combination of tetracaine, adrenaline, and cocaine (TAC) has also been shown to be an effective topical anesthetic; but it is associated with serious adverse effects (e.g., death and seizures). EMLA cream (eutectic mixture of local anesthetics) is useful, although the onset of anesthesia tends to be delayed (30–60 minutes).

Alternative agents include diphenhydramine (Benadryl) and benzyl alcohol. This is an off-label use of diphenhydramine. If diphenhydramine is used, dilute the solution to 1% to avoid tissue necrosis. Benzyl alcohol is as effective as lidocaine and is significantly less painful than injected diphenhydramine. Its duration of action is longer than that of diphenhydramine.

Regional anesthesia is recommended in cases of multiple lacerations or when large skin areas must be debrided or scrubbed (e.g., multiple imbedded glass shards, large abrasions). Since smaller volumes of anesthetic are administered, the risk of toxicity is low.

Wound Preparation

Most lacerations require primary closure. Although all traumatic lacerations should be considered contaminated, most have low bacterial counts (less than 100 microorganisms per gram of tissue). Because shaving the hair before repair may increase wound infection rates, it should be minimized. Surgical debridement of any crushed or devitalized tissue is essential because the presence of nonviable tissue may impair infection resistance. Scrubbing with a sterile surgical brush helps remove particulate matter and bacteria; but if it is done too vigorously, it can directly contribute to tissue damage and can reduce the wound's capacity to resist infection. Such damaging effects can be minimized by using a high-porosity sponge and a tissue surfactant (e.g., poloxamer 188 or Pluronic F-68). Due to high cost, their use should be reserved for highly contaminated wounds.

For irrigation, pulsatile and continuous saline are equally effective. Hydrogen peroxide, detergents, and concentrated solutions of povidone-iodine should not be used because they are toxic to tissue. Sustained high-pressure irrigation may be associated with increased tissue damage; and at very high pressures, infection rates increase. Impact irrigation pressures in the range of 5–8 psi can easily be obtained with the use of a 30- to 60-mL syringe and a 19-gauge needle or a splash shield. The latter minimizes the physician's risk of exposure to potentially infectious materials. Low-pressure irrigation is reserved for noncontaminated, highly vascular, loose areolar tissue (e.g., eyelid). Irrigation may not be required for all low-risk wounds, particularly in an area with a good vascular supply, such as the face. High-pressure irrigation is clearly indicated for lower extremity wounds. The volume of irrigation should be determined by characteristics of the wound, such as cause and location. For instance, a hand wound should be thoroughly irrigated, whereas a laceration of the eyelid requires minimal gentle irrigation.

Closure

Because the "golden period" (the time during which the benefit of closure exceeds the risk) is highly variable, each individual laceration should be considered separately. Common wound closure techniques are listed in Table 7.2. Factors, such as time of injury to presentation, infection risk, contamination, location, and cosmesis, should be weighed before the decision is made to perform primary closure. For instance, an 18-hour-old facial laceration in a child without risk factors may be closed primarily, whereas a 4-hour-old ragged dirty wound on the foot of a patient with peripheral vascular disease should not be closed primarily. Delayed primary closure after 3–5 days should be reserved for wounds with a high risk of infection.

TABLE **7.2.** Common wound closure techniques

Method	Advantages	Disadvantages
Sutures	Gold standard Lowest dehiscence rate Greatest tensile strength Meticulous closure	Anesthesia required Removal required Greatest tissue reactivity Expensive Slowest application
Staples	Quick application Inexpensive	Less meticulous closure Can interfere with computed tomography/ magnetic resonance imaging
Surgical tapes	Low cost High patient satisfaction No risk of needle stick Low reactivity Low infection rate Rapid, easy application	High rate of dehiscence Low tensile strength Must not get wet Requires use of toxic adjuncts Frequently fall off Cannot be used in areas that have large amounts of hair
Tissue adhesives	Reduced pain Reduced closure time Good cosmetic result Safe (reduced exposure to sharp needles)	Cannot use near eye or wounds with tension (across joints)

The types and characteristics of suture material are summarized in Table 7.3. The closure of the outermost layer of a laceration is done with nonabsorbable sutures, such as polypropylene and nylon, which retain most of their tensile strength for more than 60 days and which are relatively nonreactive. Generally, synthetic, monofilament sutures are preferred over natural, braided material because the infection rate is lower. Nonabsorbable sutures must be removed. Occasionally, absorbable sutures may be used to close the skin in children, thus avoiding the discomfort associated with suture removal. Closure of subcuticular structures is done with absorbable sutures. When absorbable sutures are used, 50% of a healing wound's tensile strength increases from less than 1 week to as long as 2 months. Nonsynthetic or natural absorbable suture materials, such as catgut, are more reactive and have less tensile strength than synthetic materials. Deep sutures decrease dead space and hematoma formation, relieve skin tension, and probably improve long-term cosmetic results. Liberal deep sutures that approximate skin edges should not be used in highly contaminated wounds or adipose tissue because they increase the risk of infection. Optimal results are achieved when (a) sutures are placed so that most of their tension is deep to the dermis where the connective tissue is deeper and (b) all dermal layers meet at the same level. The types of suturing techniques and their respective advantages and disadvantages are listed and illustrated in Table 7.4 and Fig. 7.1.

Staples have the following advantages: high efficacy, rapid application, and lower rates of foreign body reaction, necrosis, and infection than even the least reactive nonabsorbable suture. Staples can also be removed 1-3 days earlier than sutures. If computed tomography (CT) of the head is planned,

T ABLE 7.3.   Suture characteristics

Material	Tensile strength	Tissue reactivity	Knot security	Workability	Durability[a]	Infection risk
Absorbable						
Surgical gut (plain)	Low	High	Poor	Good	57	Low
Chromic gut	Fair	High	Low	Fair	10–14	Low
Polyglyconate (Maxon)[b]	High	Low	Fair	Excellent	45–60	Moderate
Polyglycolic acid (Dexon)	Fair	Low	Excellent	Fair	30	High
Polyglactin (Vicryl)	Fair	Low	Good	Excellent	30	High
Polydioxanone (PDS)	High	Low	Good	Good	45–60	Moderate
Nonabsorbable						
Silk	Good	High	Excellent	Excellent	>60	Fair
Nylon (Ethilon)	High	Low	Poor	Fair	>60	High
Polypropylene (Prolene)	High	Low	Poor	Fair	>60	High

[a]Maintenance of 50% tensile strength.

[b]Absorbable suture of choice.

T ABLE 7.4. Common suturing techniques

Method	Advantages	Disadvantages
Interrupted	Allows precise adjustments between sutures	Prone to cause "railroad track" eschar
Running continuous	Fast	Must remove entire suture
	Additional wound eversion	
	Even tension	
Vertical mattress	Increased wound strength	Time-consuming
	Increased wound eversion	Approximation of edges difficult
	Good dead-space closure	Removal delay associated with prominent suture marks
Buried	Approximation of wound edges	Minimal eversion
Buried vertical mattress	Prolonged eversion allows early removal of top sutures	If too superficial, suture erosion occurs
Shorthand vertical mattress	Same as vertical mattress but faster application	Edge approximation difficult
Horizontal mattress	Good wound eversion	Prone to suture scarring
	Good dead-space closure	Risk of epidermal necrosis
	Moderate hemostasis	
Subcuticular	Low incidence of scarring	Poor wound eversion
	Best for low-tension edge approximation	Time-consuming
		Poor strength under tension
Corner	Use for skin flaps because blood supply is maximized	Trauma risk
		Edge approximation difficult

closure with staples is not recommended. However, staples are more painful to remove than sutures and do not allow as meticulous a closure. The type of wound should be linear with weak skin forces.

While less reactive than staples, adhesive tapes must be used on low-tension wounds and with adhesive adjuncts (e.g., tincture of benzoin). Adhesive adjuncts increase wound infection rates and increase local induration due to tissue toxicity. They are rarely recommended for primary wound closure but are often useful after suture removal to decrease wound tension.

Tissue adhesives (e.g., 2-octylcyanoacrylates and *n*-butylcyanoacrylates) are used topically and should not be placed in the wound or between its margins. Application of three to four coats is necessary to provide adequate strength to the wound closure. Closure time and associated pain are significantly less with these products than they are with sutures, although the cosmetic result is the same. They act as their own dressing and have antimicrobial effects against gram-positive organisms. They are strongly preferred by patients and are less expensive than sutures or staples. The infection rate is less than 2%, and the dehiscence rate is 0.6%–1.8%. 2-Octylcyanoacrylate is

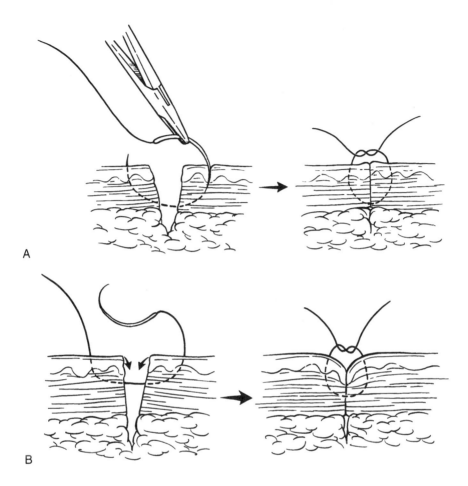

A

B

FIGURE 7.1. The skin edges should be aligned, with attention directed to the vertical axis of the incision. **A:** Optimal coaption of the skin edges occurs when the depth of suture bite and the distance from the edge of the incision are slightly greater and the bites of tissues taken on both sides of the wound are symmetrical. In deciding how the sutures should be placed, remember that, in general, the thicker the skin, the bigger the suture and the bigger the bite. For example, 3-0 sutures are placed farther from the wound edge and deeper, whereas smaller sutures are placed closer to the wound edge and not as deep. A rule of thumb is to have the needle enter the wound about halfway. **B:** A common mistake is for the suture either to be placed too far away from the edge of the incision or to be too shallow. If the suture is placed in this fashion, the skin edges will be inverted, wound healing will be compromised, and cosmesis will be suboptimal. Reprinted from Deitch EA. *Tools of the trade and rules of the road: a surgical guide.* Philadelphia, PA: Lippincott-Raven; 1997.

more stable, stronger, and more flexible than is *n*-butylcyanoacrylate. The latter is tissue toxic. Small lacerations, particularly on the face, aligned against lines of minimal tension, appear to benefit most from the use of adhesives rather than of sutures. Adhesives should not be used in lacerations that cannot be manually approximated or on skin edges that cannot be held together without significant tension. In such situations, subcutaneous or subcuticular absorbable sutures must be used to relieve tension on the skin edges. Tissue adhesives should not be used in areas that are subject to major dynamic tension or to repetitive movement (e.g., joints and hands). The adhesive usually falls off in 7-10 days as the keratinized layer of epithelium sloughs. More rapid removal can be facilitated by bathing or by the application of petroleum jelly, antibiotic ointment, or acetone.

Tetanus status should be checked, and appropriate immunization should be provided (see Table 7.1).

Antibiotics

Routine use of prophylactic antibiotics is not recommended. Decontamination of the wound site is far more important than the administration of antibiotics. However, high-risk injuries, such as certain hand wounds, cat bites, intraoral lacerations, open fractures, exposed joints or tendons, and various puncture injuries to the foot, should be treated with antibiotics. Penicillin is appropriate for cat bites (*Pasteurella* species) and hand lacerations (*Eikenella corrodens*). Tetracycline is an alternative for the penicillin-allergic patient at risk for *Pasteurella* infection. Broader coverage for these wounds can be achieved by utilizing cephalexin or a second- or third-generation cephalosporin and ampicillin-clavulinic acid combination, although these are more expensive. Penicillin is the drug of choice for intraoral lacerations. For puncture wounds of the foot, *Pseudomonas* coverage is an important consideration.

Patient Education

Because a protective nonadherent dressing should cover the wound for at least 24-48 hours until enough epithelialization has taken place to protect the wound from gross contamination, the patient should be advised to keep the wound moist, as this will speed the rate of reepithelialization. If a tissue adhesive has been used, the patient should be instructed not to apply a topical ointment and not to pick, scrub, or expose the area to excessive amounts of water since the adhesive will loosen, possibly resulting in dehiscence. After 24-48 hours, the wound should be kept clean. The patient should be instructed to report erythema, swelling, drainage, and warmth because these signs may indicate infection. The patient should also be instructed to return for staple or suture removal approximately one week later for most areas of the body. Three to five days are required for facial wounds, whereas 10-14 days are appropriate for repaired lacerations in areas of the body that are subject to high tension forces, such as the hands or joints. Patients should be told that the complete healing process takes 6–12 months and that variable amounts of redness and eschar formation will occur as the process evolves. The patient should use sunscreen on wounds exposed to prolonged sunlight to avoid hyperpigmentation during healing.

ACUTE ANGLE-CLOSURE GLAUCOMA

Glaucoma describes a group of vision disorders that share a common outcome: loss of vision secondary to optic nerve damage. Elevation of intraocular pressure (IOP), either sudden or gradual, may lead to necrosis of the nerve. The incidence of glaucoma has nearly doubled in the United States over the past 10 years to approximately 2 million. Of the various types of glaucoma, primary open-angle glaucoma is the most common, but this form is not usually associated with acute symptoms; peripheral vision is lost gradually, and central visual loss occurs late in the process. However, acute angle-closure glaucoma is associated with the sudden onset of symptoms and a high risk of vision loss if diagnosis and treatment are not prompt and appropriate.

Chief Complaint

Symptoms of acute angle-closure glaucoma include sudden onset of severe pain that affects the eye and sometimes the entire head, nausea and vomiting, blurred vision, and the perception of colored haloes around lights. Often, the eye is red. Signs include haziness of the cornea (resulting from edema of the corneal epithelium) and a nonreactive, mid-dilated pupil (4–5 mm). IOP may range from 40 to 80 mm Hg, but any pressure reading above 22 mm Hg should be taken seriously.

Pathophysiology

Acute angle-closure glaucoma accounts for as few as 10% of glaucoma cases. However, it can develop quickly; and the patient's vision may be spared only by prompt recognition and treatment. Acute angle-closure glaucoma occurs when a mid-dilated pupil obstructs the flow of aqueous humor between the posterior iris and lens. The aqueous humor accumulates in the posterior chamber and pushes the iris forward, obstructing outflow through the trabecular meshwork and producing a rise in IOP to between 40 and 70 mm Hg.

Treatment

Ultimately, acute angle-closure glaucoma is treated with laser iridectomy; however, in countries other than the United States, surgical correction of the condition may be the first step. In the United States, both topical and systemic medications are typically used as first-line therapy. In patients with an IOP of 50 mm Hg or greater, systemic osmotics may be required because, at higher pressures, the iris sphincter may not respond to topical miotic drops. Examples of systemic medications for acute, narrow-angle glaucoma include glycerol (Osmoglyn), 1.0–1.5 mL/kg orally; mannitol (Osmitrol), 12.5 g intravenously (IV); or acetazolamide (Diamox), 250–500 mg IV or orally. The particular agent that is used may depend on whether the office is equipped to administer IV medications.

When topical therapy is chosen, beta blockers (e.g., betaxolol [Betoptic], levobunolol [Betagan], timolol [Timoptic]), sympathomimetics (e.g., apraclonidine [Iopidine], brimonidine [Alphagan], dipivefrin [Propine]), or topical miotics (e.g., pilocarpine, 2% [Pilagan]) can be used. Beta blockers have been considered first-line therapy and should be given after systemic osmotics to further lower the IOP in cases of extreme elevation. The standard agent is timolol. Timolol is not cardioselective, and some systemic absorption of the beta-blocker eye solutions occurs through the nasolacrimal duct. Therefore, if cardioselectivity is desired (as in the case of a patient with asthma), the selective beta blocker betaxolol should be chosen. Not only is this agent associated with a decreased incidence of cardiac side effects, it also has been shown to be superior to timolol in preserving the visual field. Other classes of topical glaucoma agents are more likely to be used as maintenance therapy and should generally be prescribed by an ophthalmologist.

Referral

Although most family physicians' offices are not equipped for the treatment of acute angle-closure glaucoma, the family physician only needs to measure IOP with an inexpensive Schiotz tonometer to render an accurate diagnosis. A sophisticated slit lamp is not necessary. As always, the key to successful treatment is prompt recognition. Once a diagnosis has been made, the patient should quickly be referred to an ophthalmologist for prompt consultation.

OCULAR CHEMICAL BURNS

The accidental introduction of chemicals into the eye is common and requires urgent intervention. In general, these injuries produce significant damage to the ocular epithelium and cornea and, if not treated early and aggressively, may result in the permanent loss of vision.

Pathophysiology

Products containing acid or alkali are most often the cause of ocular chemical burns. Acids (e.g., battery acid, glacial acetate) cause a greater degree of ocular damage in the first few hours after exposure, but the damage is considered less progressive and penetrating than is that caused by alkali. The damage is usually localized to the area of contact, except when hydrofluoric acid or heavy metal is involved, in which case the damage is more extensive.

Alkaline burns, such as those caused by lime, lye, potassium hydroxide, magnesium hydroxide, and ammonia, are more severe than acid burns because the corneal epithelium is rapidly penetrated. Lysis of the cell membranes occurs, and the damage is often permanent. The extent of ocular injury is related to the concentration of the chemical and to the time elapsed between injury and treatment. When in doubt, injuries caused by other chemicals, such as mace, tear gas, flares, and sparklers, should be treated as alkaline burns.

Treatment

Lavage of the affected eye should begin immediately, using whatever water is readily available, and should continue for several minutes. After this has been done, the patient should be transferred to an emergency department for continued lavage. If transfer to an emergency department is not feasible, continue lavage and perform frequent (every 5-10 minutes) checks of the ocular pH with litmus paper. Continue lavage with 2 L of normal saline for at least an hour or until the ocular pH is in the range of 7.3-7.7.

When the pH has reached the normal range and remains stable, mydriatic/cycloplegic drops, such as 5% homatropine or 1% cyclopentolate, should be used to prevent adhesions and spasm. Topical antibiotics (e.g., gentamicin, bacitracin, erythromycin) are given to prevent infection. Burns caused by alkaline chemicals can produce a rapid rise in IOP as the sclera constricts. To prevent this, give carbonic anhydrase inhibitors, such as acetazolamide (Diamox), 500 mg, immediately by IV or by mouth and then give 250 mg by mouth three times a day. Topical steroids should be used only in the first 7-10 days following injury and should then be stopped to prevent interference with the stromal repair process.

A chemical burn in the eye is exquisitely painful, and the process of lavage is likely to produce significant anxiety for the patient. Besides ocular anesthetic drops, narcotic pain medication and/or anxiolytic medications should be used. The physician must also remember that the upper airway may also have been burned or compromised, and a careful examination of this area should be undertaken while the patient is in the office. Because of the intense pain and anxiety associated with these burns and the risk of upper airway compromise, patients who have sustained an ocular chemical burn should be transferred to the nearest emergency department by ambulance once they are stable.

Prognosis

Ocular chemical burns can be classified as mild, moderate, or severe based on the appearance of the cornea. The less opacification and scarring that is seen, the better the prognosis is. Severe burns, in which the cornea is opalescent, the epithelium is absent, and the pupil is obscured with external "whitening," are associated with the poorest prognosis for preservation of vision.

CENTRAL RETINAL ARTERY OCCLUSION

Occlusion of the central retinal artery is a true emergency that often results in permanent vision loss. Even a 2-hour delay in treatment may result in vision loss.

Chief Complaint

Patients with central retinal artery occlusion complain of a sudden onset of painless total loss of vision and light perception. An afferent pupillary defect exists. On ophthalmoscopy, a "cherry-red" spot is seen on the macula.

Pathophysiology

Embolization from the major arteries supplying the head or from the left side of the heart can cause central retinal artery occlusion. Blood supply to the retina is then obstructed with resulting infarction of the inner two-thirds of the retina. Blood flow must be reestablished within 90 minutes. Risk factors include coronary artery disease, connective tissue disorders (e.g., giant cell arteritis), sickle cell anemia, and syphilis.

Treatment

Although attempts to restore the patient's vision may be futile if the occlusion has been present for more than 2 hours, such attempts should be made for symptoms of even 2 days' duration. Immediate ophthalmologic consultation should be sought; but in the interim, ballottement of the globe (i.e., intermittent digital pressure for 5–30 minutes) should be performed. Inhalation of a 95% oxygen/5% carbon dioxide mixture, intravenous acetazolamide, and paracentesis of aqueous humor from the anterior chamber may increase blood flow, dislodge emboli from the artery, and dilate the retinal vasculature.

EPISTAXIS

Nosebleed, or epistaxis, is fairly common and will affect 11% of the general population at some point. Common causes include upper airway inflammation, such as that caused by infections of the nose and throat, rhinitis medicamentosa, and allergic rhinitis. Trauma, including that which results from surgery or the presence of foreign bodies (including the index finger), can also cause significant epistaxis. Furthermore, systemic illness, such as hypertension and coronary artery disease, liver failure, coagulopathies and other hematologic conditions, and renal disease, often predispose a patient to bouts of epistaxis. Many common prescription medications (e.g., acetylsalicylic acid, anticoagulants) and recreational drugs (e.g., cocaine) can also predispose patients to epistaxis.

Pathophysiology

The blood supply to the nose comes from the internal and external carotid arteries. The most likely site of an anterior nasal bleed is the part of the nasal septum known as Little's area, where an anastomosis of several arterioles—anterior ethmoid, sphenopalatine, greater palatine, and superior labial—known as Kiesselbach's plexus exists. Posterior nosebleeds may only account for 5% of all cases and commonly involve the lateral nasal branch of the sphenopalatine artery. Young patients and otherwise healthy adults tend to have more anterior bleeds, whereas the elderly are more likely to experience epistaxis from a posterior source.

Diagnosis

Initially, the site of bleeding must be identified. Adequate lighting, including a headlamp if available, and a suction-tip or Yankauer-style catheter to remove blood and clots are essential. Have the patient apply compression for 10 minutes by squeezing the nose between the proximal interphalangeal and distal interphalangeal joints of the index finger and the thumb. A vasoconstrictor (such as epinephrine 1:1,000 or a 4% solution of cocaine on a pledget or oxymetazoline spray [Afrin, Dristan, etc.]) combined with a local anesthetic will help to control the bleeding long enough to identify the site. If the bleeding has stopped, the site is likely anterior; and no further treatment is necessary, although the patient should be observed for a short time to see if relapse occurs. However, if bleeding is still evident, is bilateral, or is trickling down the throat, the site is more likely to be posterior.

Treatment

Anterior Epistaxis

Treatment of anterior epistaxis is easily accomplished by the use of chemical cautery, silver nitrate sticks, or 25% tetrocaine, cocaine, adrenaline (TCA) if the site is readily identifiable. Thermal cautery with hand-held or Bovie instrumentation is not advised as even a minor slip can result in perforation of the nasal septum. If local measures are ineffective, anterior nasal packs should be placed to tamponade the bleeding. Such packs can be constructed with petrolatum gauze; commercially available anterior nasal packs (e.g., Merocel nasal tampon) are convenient and effective. Antibiotics effective against *Staphylococcus aureus* should be given to every patient who has a nasal packing to guard against infection. Anterior nasal packs should be removed by an otolaryngologist.

Posterior Epistaxis

Treatment of this disorder is more difficult and time-consuming than is treatment of anterior epistaxis. In the past, posterior packs were constructed with gauze and silk ties, but this is time-consuming. Commercially made posterior packs (Nasostat epistaxis balloon, Storz epistaxis catheter) use balloons to tamponade the bleeding artery. If these are not readily available, a 12- to 16-Fr Foley catheter with the balloon inflated with 5 mL of water is effective. These devices, resembling a nasal trumpet, are placed in the nasal cavity through one of the nares; when in place, the balloons are inflated with normal saline using a syringe. However, placement of posterior tamponading devices is painful; and, in fact, unless the patient feels an uncomfortable pressure in the nasal, sinus, and pharyngeal areas, the pack is not placed properly. Such packs may produce hypoxia, which can lead to cardiac disturbances and can result in necrosis of the nasal structures. For these reasons, patients with posterior epistaxis should be admitted to the hospital, even if the posterior bleed is controlled; and a search for the cause should be initiated.

If the bleeding is still not controlled, several surgical and nonsurgical techniques may be employed to stop the hemorrhage. Identification of the bleeding site with digital subtraction angiography may be utilized. Transarterial embolization with gelatin sponges, collagen, or polyvinyl alcohol carries a high success rate in treating severe epistaxis. Endoscopic cauterization has also been effective and has a success rate of 90%. It is associated with less morbidity than surgical ligation. In cases of severe, intractable epistaxis, surgical ligation may be the only way to control bleeding.

TOOTH AVULSION

Chief Complaint

Displacement of a tooth out of the oral cavity is found.

Diagnosis

The patient's age should be determined first, as primary teeth do not need to be reimplanted. Determine whether significant head trauma has also occurred, and treat accordingly. The mechanism of injury is an important piece of history to obtain.

Treatment

If the patient cannot be seen by a dental professional immediately, instruct the patient (or parent) to hold the tooth by the crown only, never to touch the root, and to rinse dirt off without scrubbing. Avulsed teeth should be stored in milk or wet gauze until the patient can be seen. The patient should not carry the tooth in his or her mouth; replacing a completely avulsed tooth into a socket, without fixation, significantly increases the likelihood of aspiration.

Referral

Ideally, the tooth should be replaced and fixated in the socket by a dental specialist as soon as possible (within 2–3 hours) because the likelihood of successful reimplantation decreases by one percentage point for each minute the tooth is out of the oral cavity. If the tooth is only partially avulsed, replace it in position with digital pressure; recommend a diet of soft foods; and refer the patient to a dentist immediately.

ACUTE ABDOMEN

The hallmark of an acute abdomen is pain. Typically, the patient's description of the pain will differ depending on the condition. For example, severe, explosive pain suggests a ruptured vascular or hollow viscus (e.g., abdominal aortic aneurysm or ectopic pregnancy rupture). Rapidly worsening pain is consistent with pancreatitis, mesenteric ischemia, and strangulation of the small bowel. Peritoneal inflammation causes pain that is duller, more vague, and more gradual in nature; pain that does not resolve with narcotics may be caused by vascular compromise. Colicky pain indicates gastroenteritis, cholelithiasis, or nephrolithiasis. Referred pain to the shoulder suggests splenic, hepatic, or gall bladder disease; if referred to the back, it may indicate renal pathology; that referred to the groin may signify renal or hernia problems.

Chief Complaint

No set clinical course for acute abdominal pain exists; patients may report that their symptoms began weeks or just minutes prior to their arrival in the office. Besides pain, associated symptoms, such as anorexia, nausea, vomiting, fever, or vaginal spotting (in the female patient), may be present.

Diagnosis

On physical examination, note the patient's body position, skin turgor, and the presence of abdominal distention. Signs of the acute abdomen include tenderness on palpation, involuntary guarding of the abdominal muscles, rebound tenderness, and hypoactive bowel sounds.

Auscultation of bowel sounds in all four quadrants is key. The abdominal wall should be palpated for rectus spasm and should be percussed to determine bladder distention, ascites, and costovertebral angle tenderness. Every patient should have a rectal or stomal examination, and stool should be tested for occult blood. Female patients require a pelvic examination, both bimanual and using a speculum, to rule out genitourinary and pelvic disorders. Table 7.5 lists differential diagnoses to consider in the patient with an acute abdomen.

Testing

Diagnostic tests may help confirm a diagnosis but should not take the place of surgical consultation and/or admission for observation. Laboratory evalu-

T ABLE 7.5. Common causes of acute abdominal pain

Inflammatory
Appendicitis
Diverticulitis
Cholecystitis
Perforated peptic ulcer
Acute pancreatitis
Obstructive
Adhesions
Hernia
Intussusception
Volvulus
Diverticular disease
Cancer
Vascular
Mesenteric ischemia
Ruptured abdominal aortic aneurysm
Genitourinary
Urinary tract infection
Kidney stone
Dysmenorrhea
Ectopic pregnancy
Pelvic inflammatory disease

ation consists of complete blood count with differential, electrolytes, amylase, urinalysis, and appropriate cultures. A serum pregnancy test is essential for females. Radiographic studies include upright chest x-ray to evaluate for free air; flat-plate abdomen to assess gas, peritoneal fat lines, and psoas shadow; ultrasonography to detect gallstones and ectopic pregnancy (females); intravenous pyelography to evaluate kidney stones and masses; and barium enema to rule out suspected intussusception, diverticulitis, and appendicitis.

Treatment

Whereas the ultimate treatment of the acute abdomen may involve surgical exploration, the family physician must maintain a high index of suspicion and must differentiate between patients who are likely to require immediate surgery and those who may only require observation. If appropriate, start IV fluids and antibiotics. Analgesia, with short-acting narcotics, should be used judiciously to alleviate distress but should not interfere with the diagnostic process.

Referral

The patient should be admitted, and surgical consult should obtained sooner rather than later. With this in mind, ensure that the patient takes nothing (food or medications) by mouth.

PARAPHIMOSIS

A true urologic emergency, paraphimosis occurs when a tight foreskin cannot advance past the corona of the glans penis. The glans becomes edematous, making the replacement of the foreskin more difficult; this can result in arterial compromise and gangrene. Risk factors for paraphimosis include a localized, mild phimosis and the presence of an indwelling urinary catheter in uncircumcised men.

Treatment

When replacing the foreskin, local anesthesia with lidocaine (via a dorsal penile nerve block) may be needed. Compression of the glans and distal penis may be adequate to advance the foreskin; but if not, then a dorsal vertical slit of the compressing band is necessary. Recurrent bouts of paraphimosis are an indication for circumcision.

TESTICULAR TORSION

Testicular torsion is not merely a urologic emergency; it is a potential surgical emergency as well. It occurs secondary to an incomplete reflection of the tunica vaginalis on the testis and epididymis, allowing the testis to freely rotate inside the tunica. This rotation can result in strangulation of the blood supply to the organ.

Chief Complaint

The pain associated with testicular torsion is not positional—as is the case with epididymitis, where elevation helps—and it may be accompanied by nausea and vomiting. Clinically, the testis is typically swollen, is markedly tender, and is situated more superiorly and transversely than is the contralateral testis.

Epidemiologic Factors

Although testicular torsion can occur at any age, the peak incidence is at puberty. Frequently, the patient has a history of athletic activity prior to onset; however, in adolescents, no apparent risk factors commonly exist, and boys may simply report waking from sleep with an acute pain in the scrotum.

Diagnosis

The consequences of a missed testicular torsion are dire: if the diagnosis is not made promptly and blood flow to the testicle is not restored within hours, the chances of salvaging the testicle are slim. Therefore, in the patient with acute testicular pain, rule out torsion first. Suspicion warrants an immediate urologic consultation. The differential diagnosis includes epididymitis, hernia, and torsion of the testicular appendage. The incidence of torsion in the setting of acute scrotal edema may only be about 25%.

Testing

Confirmatory tests include urinalysis, complete blood cell count, and testicular ultrasonography. Typically, a 4-hour window of opportunity (beginning at the onset of pain) exists for salvaging the testicle. Thus, surgical exploration should not be delayed to wait for the results of ultrasonographic imaging.

Treatment

Detorsion, in a medial-to-lateral direction and with the use of local anesthesia, should be attempted while awaiting surgical exploration.

Prognosis

Both the patient and the physician should keep in mind that the other testis has a higher than average incidence of recurrence.

ACUTE COMPARTMENT SYNDROME

Acute compartment syndrome describes a condition in which increased tissue pressure within a closed space compromises the vital circulatory and neural structures within that space. Normal tissue pressure is usually 0–10 mm Hg, and capillary blood flow to the nerves and muscle decreases when pressure exceeds 20 mm Hg. Although arterial flow is not compromised at these pressures, ischemic necrosis of muscle and nerve tissue occurs when the pressures exceed 30–40 mm Hg. Thus, although distal pulses are still palpable, considerable damage may result if an acute compartment syndrome is not suspected and treatment is not initiated.

Chief Complaint

The clinical signs and symptoms of acute compartment syndrome worsen with time. Initially, the patient will report pain out of proportion to the perceived injury. The pain is exacerbated by active contraction and passive stretching of the involved muscles. As tissue pressures increase, pain progresses to muscle weakness; although muscles are more sensitive to ischemia than nerves, actual motor deficits may be a later finding. Paresthesia and anesthesia, which are decreases in nerve sensation, indicate neural ischemia.

Unless an artery has been damaged, peripheral pulses rarely are absent until the pressure in the compartment has risen above the patient's diastolic blood pressure. Thus, discounting the possibility of a compartment syndrome based on the presence of a distal pulse may result in a missed diagnosis and, ultimately, in irreversible neuromuscular damage to the limb.

Pathophysiology

The etiology of compartment syndrome is fairly straightforward: anything that causes the size of a fascial compartment to decrease or that causes the compartment contents to increase puts the patient at risk. For example, constrictive dressings, such as casts and bandages, can decrease the size of a compartment, whereas edema or hemorrhage can increase the contents of a compartment. Factors commonly associated with compartment syndrome include frostbite, arterial injury and vasospasm, limb immobilization and compression, animal bites, fractures, surgery, ruptured popliteal cysts, and the use of medications containing ergotamines.

Diagnosis

Prompt recognition of compartment syndrome is the cornerstone of proper treatment. Pressures within fascial compartments can be measured using battery-powered monitors. However, most family physicians do not have these devices in their offices, so the diagnosis usually is based on a high index of suspicion.

Treatment

Any constrictive dressings or casts should be removed immediately. Because incision, drainage, or fasciotomy may be required to save the extremity, emergent surgical consultation is necessary. The family physician should attempt these procedures in the office only if considerable delay in reaching a surgeon is likely; even then, the procedures should only be done by physicians properly trained in their implementation. For pressures in the range of 15–20 mm Hg, the patient may be observed, and repeat measurements should be taken if symptoms fail to improve. Any reading over 20 mm Hg requires admission and surgical consultation; and if pressures exceed 30 mm Hg, emergency fasciotomy by longitudinal incision over the compartment must be undertaken to avoid irreversible compromise.

REFERENCES

1. Alvi A, Joyner-Triplett N. Acute epistaxis: how to spot the source and stop the flow. *Postgrad Med* 1996;99(5):83–96.

2. Chaudhry I, Wong S. Recognizing glaucoma: a guide for the primary care physician. *Postgrad Med* 1996;99(5):247–264.

3. Dawson C, Whitfield H. Urological emergencies in general practice. *BMJ* 1996; 312:838–840.

4. Epstein DL, Pavan-Langston D. Glaucoma. In: Pavan-Langston D, ed. *Manual of ocular diagnosis and therapy,* 2nd ed. Boston: Little, Brown and Co., 1985:201–229.

5. Fales WD, Overton DT. Abdominal pain. In: Tintinalli JE, Ruiz E, Krome RL, eds. *Emergency medicine: a comprehensive study guide,* 4th ed. New York: McGraw-Hill, 1996:217–221.

6. Janda AM. Ocular emergencies. In: Tintinalli JE, Ruiz E, Krome RL, eds. *Emergency medicine: a comprehensive study guide,* 4th ed. New York: McGraw-Hill, 1996:1066.

7. Kini MM. Retina and vitreous. In: Pavan-Langston D, ed. *Manual of ocular diagnosis and therapy,* 2nd ed. Boston: Little, Brown and Co., 1985:148.

8. Lewis PR, Phillips TG, Sassani JW. Topical therapies for glaucoma: what family physicians need to know. *Am Fam Physician* 1999;59:1871–1879.

9. Linehan WM. The urogenital system. In: Sabiston DE, ed. *Essentials of surgery.* Philadelphia: WB Saunders, 1987:851.

10. Margarone JE, Hall R. Management of alveolar and dental fractures. In: Peterson LJ, ed. *Principles of oral and maxillofacial surgery.* Philadelphia: JB Lippincott, 1992:396.

11. Martin RF, Rossi RL. The acute abdomen: an overview and algorithms. *Surg Clin N Am* 1997;77(6):1227–1242.

12. Merland JJ, Fox RB, Rogers AK. Place of embolization in the treatment of severe epistaxis. *Laryngoscope* 1980;90(10):1694–1704.

13. Morris JA, Sawyers JL. The acute abdomen. In: Sabiston DE, ed. *Essentials of surgery.* Philadelphia: WB Saunders, 1987:388–405.

14. Pavan-Langston D. Burns and trauma. In: Pavan-Langston D, ed. *Manual of ocular diagnosis and therapy,* 2nd ed. Boston: Little, Brown and Co., 1985:31–33.

15. Ruiz E. Compartment syndromes. In: Tintinalli JE, Ruiz E, Krome RL, eds. *Emergency medicine: a comprehensive study guide,* 4th ed. New York: McGraw-Hill, 1996:1307–1311.

16. Schneider RE. Male genital problems. In: Tintinalli JE, Ruiz E, Krome RL, eds. *Emergency medicine: a comprehensive study guide,* 4th ed. New York: McGraw-Hill, 1996:536.

17. Smith JA. Epistaxis. In: Tintinalli JE, Ruiz E, Krome RL, eds. *Emergency medicine: a comprehensive study guide,* 4th ed. New York: McGraw-Hill, 1996: 1082–1087.

18. Tarraza HM, Moore RD. Gynecologic causes of the acute abdomen and the acute abdomen in pregnancy. *Surg Clin N Am* 1997;77:1371-1394.

19. Van Essen GJ, McQueen MM. Compartment syndrome in the lower limb. *Hosp Med* 1998;59(4):294-297.

20. Viducich RA, Blanda MP, Gerson LW. Posterior epistaxis: clinical features and acute complications. *Ann Emerg Med* 1995;25:592-596.

21. Wagoner MD. Chemical injuries of the eye: current concepts in pathophysiology and therapy. *Survey Ophthalmol* 1997;41:275-312.

22. Willis RB, Rorabeck CH. Treatment of compartment syndrome in children. *Orthop Clin N Am* 1990;21:401-412.

23. Singer AJ, Hollander JE, Quinn JV. Evaluation and management of traumatic lacerations. *N Engl J Med* 1997;337:1142-1148.

24. Browne EZ. Wound suturing: achieving optimal results. *Mod Med* 1987; 55(5):46-48.

25. Whealton EG. Advances in office anesthesia. *J Am Board Fam Pract* 1998;11(3):200-206.

26. Moy RL, Lee A, Zalka A. Commonly used suturing techniques in skin surgery. *Am Fam Physician* 1991;44(5):1625-1634.

27. Moy RL, Lee A, Zalka A. Commonly used suture materials in skin surgery. *Am Fam Physician* 1991;44(6):2123-2128.

CHAPTER 8

....

Infectious

Shaikh Hasan and Richard B. Birrer

MENINGITIS

Meningitis is a disease of the central nervous system (CNS) that involves inflammation of the meninges, the three membranes of the brain or spinal cord. The etiologies are classified as infectious (e.g., bacteria, viruses, fungi, parasites, tuberculosis) and noninfectious (e.g., neoplastic, collagen-vascular) (Table 8.1).

Chief Complaint

A concerned mother brings her 10-week-old daughter to the office. The girl is irritable and febrile, has been vomiting and is not breast-feeding well. She has missed some of her vaccinations.

A 48-year-old man presents for an emergency sick visit. Symptoms include generalized headache (new onset), intractable vomiting, fever, nuchal rigidity, photophobia, and a change in baseline mental status.

Clinical Manifestations

The signs and symptoms of meningitis are numerous (Table 8.2). Classic cases provide little diagnostic challenge: the patient presents with fever, severe headache, stiff neck, photophobia, and altered mental status. The clinical challenge is seen in the very young and the elderly in whom the presenting symptoms might be incomplete and nonspecific. Approximately 75% of patients with bacterial meningitis present with subacute symptoms.

The physical findings in meningitis vary, depending on the severity of the illness, host factors, and causative organisms. Nuchal rigidity, Brudzinski's sign, and Kernig's sign are seen in approximately 50% of adults.

- *Kernig's sign:* The patient can easily and completely extend the leg when in dorsal decubitus position but not when in the sitting posture or when lying with the thigh flexed on the abdomen.
- *Brudzinski's sign:* Flexion of the neck usually results in flexion of the hip and knee; when passive flexion of the lower limb on one side is carried out, a similar movement can be seen in the opposite limb.

T ABLE 8.1. Infectious and noninfectious causes

Bacterial	Fungal
Streptococcus pneumoniae	*Cryptococcus meningitidis*
Neisseria meningitidis	*Coccidioides*
Listeria monocytogenes	*Candida*
Haemophilus influenzae	*Blastomyces*
Staphylococcus aureus	*Histoplasma*
Streptococci	**Noninfectious**
Koch bacilli	Carcinomatous meningitis
Mycobacterium tuberculosis	Systemic lupus erythematosus
Viral	Vasculitis
Herpes simplex viruses	Sarcoidosis
Epstein–Barr virus	Serum sickness
Cytomegalovirus	Chemical meningitis (nonsteroidals, isoniazid, and
Varicella-zoster virus	trimethoprim)
Human immunodeficiency virus	
Arboviruses	
Human T-cell leukemia/lymphoma virus	

Integumentary examination may reveal a meningococcemia rash, initially with macular and erythematous changes, which may transition into petechiae, splinter hemorrhages, or pustular lesions.

Funduscopic examination may reveal papilledema, which presents in only one-third of meningitis patients, with increased intracranial pressure that develops over several hours.

T ABLE 8.2. Signs and symptoms of meningitis

Bacterial	Viral
Antecedent upper respiratory infection	Fever
Fever	Headache, often sudden
Headache	Stiff neck
Meningism	Nausea and vomiting
Photophobia	Photophobia
Seizures	Generalized aches and pains
Nausea	Occasional rash
Rigors	
Weakness	
Altered mental status	
Focal neurologic deficits	

Epidemiologic Factors

The incidence of bacterial meningitis is 5–10 cases per 100,000 persons per year. The disease may occur at any time of the year, but its incidence increases in late winter and early spring.

The incidence of viral meningitis is 15–30 cases per 100,000 persons per year. It is prominently seen in summer.

Risk Factors

Numerous host factors have been implicated (Table 8.3).

Age

The relative frequency of various species as a cause of meningitis varies with age (Table 8.4). Patients younger than 5 years of age or older than 60 years are at higher risk. Approximately 400 out of 100,000 neonates and only 1 or 2 out of 100,000 adults will acquire meningitis.

Race

Navajo Indian and American Eskimo populations may have genetic or acquired vulnerability to this invasive disease.

Region

Meningococcal meningitis is endemic in parts of Africa.

Sex

A higher incidence is noted in men than in women.

T ABLE 8.3.   Host factors predisposing to meningitis

Age >60 yr	Diabetes
Intravenous drug abuse	Recent colonization
Male sex	Dural defect (e.g., traumatic, surgical, congenital)
Alcoholism and cirrhosis	Contiguous infection (e.g., sinusitis)
Low socioeconomic status	Immunocompromised status
Household contact	Thalassemia major
Bacterial endocarditis	Malignancy (increased risk for *Listeria* infection)
African-American	Splenectomy (increased risk for encapsulated organisms)
Ventriculoperitoneal shunt	

Sickle cell disease (increased risk for encapsulated organisms)
Crowding (e.g., military recruits), increased risk for meningococcal meningitis
Age <5 yr (especially with diabetes, renal or adrenal insufficiency, hypoparathyroidism, and cystic fibrosis)

TABLE 8.4. Bacterial etiologic agents of meningitis, by patient age (%)

Organism	Neonates (<1 mo)	Children (1 mo to 15 yr)	Adults (>15 yr)
H. influenzae	0–3	40–60	1–3
S. pneumoniae	0–5	10–20	30–50
N. meningitidis	0–1	25–40	10–35
Gram-negative bacilli	50–60	1–2	1–10
Streptococci	20–40[a]	2–4	5
Staphylococci	5	1–2	5–15
Listeria species	2–10	1–2	5

[a]Nearly all isolates are group B streptococci.

Pathophysiology

Histologic changes vary according to the stage of the disease and the associated organisms. Bacterial meningitis consists of exudative accumulation within the subarachnoid space extending to the spinal cord and nerve sheaths in the absence of obstruction. A number of factors influence the development of bacterial meningitis, including virulence of the strain, host defenses, and bacteria–host interactions. Bacterial cell wall components initiate a cascade of complement and cytokine-mediated events, which results in cerebral edema, presence of toxic mediators in the cerebral spinal fluid (CSF), and increased blood–brain barrier permeability. As intracranial pressure increases, brain edema progresses, leading to failure of the autoregulatory process and to decreased cerebral blood flow (CBF). This causes ischemic injury and eventually leads to systemic complications. Lymphocytic pleocytosis is the typical finding in viral meningitis. Subintimal infiltration of arterial walls by lymphocytes and neutrophils is relatively unique to infection of the meninges.

Diagnosis

The clinical presentation is distinctive and sufficient in the classical presentation (Table 8.2). Meningitis should be considered in every patient with fever, an altered mental status, and other meningeal signs and symptoms.

The differential diagnoses are listed in Table 8.5.

Diagnostic Tests

Lumbar Puncture

Definitive diagnosis is based on examination of the CSF (Table 8.6). Deferring lumbar puncture until a computed tomography (CT) scan has been obtained may be necessary for patients with clinical evidence of papilledema, intracranial mass, recent-onset seizure, head trauma, or focal neurologic deficit.

T ABLE 8.5. Differential diagnoses of meningitis

Bacteremia/sepsis
Brain abscess
Seizures
Acute encephalopathy
Postinfectious encephalomyelitis
Parameningeal infections (e.g., subdural empyema)
Carcinomatous meningitis
Migraine headache
Meningeal leukemia
Drug-induced meningitis

Neuroimaging Studies

These are indicated in any patient with symptoms compatible with CNS infections or abscess.

Additional Testing

Complete blood count with differential, electrolytes to evaluate for dehydration or syndrome of inappropriate antidiuretic hormone (SIADH), urine, and nasopharyngeal cultures are commonly used; blood cultures (two specimens drawn 15 minutes apart) may also be taken.

Referral

The family physician can adequately treat meningitis. Patients with suspected bacterial meningitis should be placed in the intensive care setting with appropriate isolation protocol. For patients with multiple complications, such as

T ABLE 8.6. Typical spinal fluid results for meningeal processes

Parameter (normal)	Bacterial	Viral	Neoplastic	Fungal
OP (<170 mm CSF)	>300 mm	200 mm	200 mm	300 mm
WBC (<5 mononuclear)	>1,000/μL	<1,000/μL	<500/μL	<500/μL
% PMNS (0)	>80%	1–50%	1–50%	1–50%
Glucose (>40 mg/dL)	<40 mg/dL	>40 mg/dL	<40 mg/dL	<40 mg/dL
Protein (<50 mg/dL)	>200 mg/dL	<200 mg/dL	>200 mg/dL	>200 mg/dL
Gram stain (−)	(+)	(−)	(−)	(−)
Cytology (−)	(−)	(−)	(+)	(+)

CSF, cerebrospinal fluid; OP, opening pressure; PMNS, polymorphonuclear cells; WBC, white blood cells.

shock, disseminated intravascular coagulation, and so forth, consultation with a critical care physician and infectious disease specialist may be warranted.

Management

The family physician must remember that only early recognition and treatment decrease the incidence of death and serious disability from meningitis.

Bacterial Meningitis (Table 8.7)

Until the organism is identified, broad-spectrum coverage is required. Initial empirical therapy usually consists of ampicillin and cefotaxime (Claforan) within 30 minutes of presentation. Once the pathogen is isolated, antimicrobial therapy can be modified on the basis of susceptibility.

Controversy surrounds the use of dexamethasone (Decadron). It is thought to interrupt the cytokine-mediated neurotoxic effects of bacterioly-

T ABLE 8.7. Treatment regimens for bacterial meningitis

Age	Potential pathogens	Initial empirical therapy
Full-term Neonates		
Neonate (0–7 days)	Group B *Streptococcus, Listeria monocytogenes,* aerobic gram-negative bacilli	Cefotaxime (Claforan), 50 mg/kg IV every 12 hr, plus ampicillin, 100 mg/kg IV every 12 hrs; orampicillin, 100 mg/kg IV every 12 hr, plus gentamicin, 2.5 mg/kg IV every 12 hr
Neonate (8–28 days)	As above	Cefotaxime, 50 mg/kg IV every 8 hr, plus ampicillin, 100 mg/kg IV every 8 hr
Infants and Adults		
Infants (1–3 months)	Group B *Streptococcus, Listeria monocytogenes, Haemophilus influenzae, Streptococcus pneumoniae, Neisseria meningitidis*	Cefotaxime, 50 mg/kg IV every 6 hr, plus ampicillin, 200–400 mg/kg/d divided every 4–6 hrs
3 months–18 years	*Haemophilus influenzae, Streptococcus pneumoniae, Neisseria meningitidis*	Ceftriaxone (Rocephin), 80–100 mg/kg/d divided every 12–24 hr (not to exceed 4 g/24 hr), or cefotaxime, 50 mg/kg IV every 6 hr (not to exceed 12 g/24 hr)
18–50 years	*Streptococcus pneumoniae, Neisseria meningitidis*	Ceftriaxone, 2 g IV every 12 hr
Older than 50 years	*Streptococcus pneumoniae, Haemophilus influenzae, Listeria monocytogenes,* aerobic gram-negative bacilli	Ceftriaxone, 2 g IV every 12 hr, plus ampicillin, 2 g IV every 4 hr

sis, which are maximal during the first few days of antibiotic use. Its use has mostly been in the pediatric population; adult studies have been limited and inadequate. The U.S. Food and Drug Administration has not approved its use for the treatment of bacterial meningitis.

Viral Meningitis

No specific treatment is available for viral meningitis other than for herpes simplex virus (HSV) meningitis. The agent of choice for HSV is intravenous acyclovir (Zovirax). Supportive therapy is required because the infection is usually benign and self-limiting. When doubt exists as to the possibility of a bacterial cause, appropriate antimicrobial therapy should be initiated; and a repeat lumbar puncture should be performed within 8–12 hours.

Pediatric Cases

Dexamethasone, 0.15 mg per kilogram per dose, given intravenously every 6 hours for 2 days, is recommended for infants and children 6 weeks or older with strongly suspected bacterial meningitis. Clinical trials confirm decreased morbidity, especially decreased incidence and severity of neurosensory hearing loss, for *Haemophilus influenzae* meningitis and suggest comparable benefit for *Staphylococcus pneumoniae* meningitis in childhood.

Follow-up

Potential problems and complications are listed in Table 8.8.

Infants with bacterial meningitis should have a brain-stem auditory evoked response (BAER) test performed prior to hospital discharge.

T ABLE 8.8. Possible complications of meningitis

Bacterial
Seizures (20%–30% during course of illness)
Focal neurologic deficit
Sensorineural hearing loss (10% risk in children)
Subdural effusions
Obstructive hydrocephalus
Neurodevelopmental sequelae (30% risk of subtle learning deficits)
Cranial nerve palsies (III, VI, VII, VIII) (10%–20% of cases, usually disappear within a few weeks)
Viral
Deafness
Fatigue
Irritability
Muscle weakness
Seizures (rare)

Repeat lumbar puncture is not necessary in viral meningitis unless the clinical course is atypical.

Prevention

The American College Health Association (ACHA) recommends that physicians offer college-bound students vaccination against meningococcal disease. However, the American Academy of Family Physicians (AAFP) states that physicians need not initiate discussion of this vaccine as part of routine medical care given the large number of issues that are of greater importance in the care of young adults. The AAFP policy also states that colleges may provide education on meningococcal infection and vaccination and may offer it to those who are interested.

Prophylaxis is indicated for those at increased risk, such as those in close contact with the patient for at least 4 hours during the week before onset (e.g., housemates, day care center mates, cell mates) or those exposed to the patient's nasopharyngeal secretions (e.g., via kissing, mouth-to-mouth resuscitation, intubation, and nasotracheal suctioning).

Adult patients with meningococcal meningitis exposure should be given rifampin (Rifadin), 600 mg orally every 12 hours for 2 days. Children younger than 12 months with *H. influenzae* meningitis exposure should receive rifampin, 10 mg per kg every 12 hours for 2 days. The physician should note that rifampin only eradicates the organism from the nasopharynx and is ineffective against invasive disease. Instruct all contacts to be evaluated immediately at the first sign of fever, sore throat, rash, or symptoms of meningitis. Possible therapeutic alternatives include ciprofloxacin (Cipro), 500 mg orally in a single dose (an off-label use), or a single intramuscular dose of ceftriaxone (Rocephin), 125 mg for patients younger than 15 years or 250 mg for older patients.

Patient Education

Educational materials on meningitis may be obtained by contacting the American Academy of Pediatrics by phone at (847) 434-4000 or on the Web at www.aap.org.

SEPSIS AND SEPTIC SHOCK

Sepsis and septic shock are clinical syndromes that result from acute invasion of the blood by certain microorganisms and/or their toxic products. Patients with sepsis usually have a fever, tachycardia, tachypnea, leukocytosis, and a localized site of infection, although 20% of elderly patients may not present with such signs. When this syndrome results in hypotension or multiple organ system failure, the condition is called septic shock.

Chief Complaint

A 35-year-old woman presents to the office with a 1-day history of cough, fever, and shaking chills. She has suffered from upper respiratory symptoms for the past 2 days. Her past medical history is significant for systemic lupus erythematosus, for which she takes low-dose prednisone. Physical examination reveals that she is in acute distress. Her pulse is 120 beats per minute; blood pressure, 90/55 mm Hg; respiratory rate, 24/min; and temperature, 104.1°F. Chest examination reveals bilateral rates and decreased breath sounds on the right side. Chest x-ray confirms bilateral pneumonia.

Etiologic Factors

Gram-negative and gram-positive organisms and fungi can cause sepsis and septic shock. Certain viruses and rickettsiae probably can produce a similar syndrome. *Escherichia coli, Klebsiella enterobacter, Proteus, Pseudomonas,* and *Serratia* are the most common gram-negative bacteria and are present in 60%–70% percent of cases. Staphylococci, pneumococci, streptococci, and other gram-positive organisms are less frequent causes and are responsible for 20%–40% percent of cases. Frequently, the origins of sepsis can be traced to pyelonephritis, pneumonia, peritonitis, cholangitis, cellulitis, meningitis, or abscess formation at any site. Many of these infections are nosocomial.

Epidemiologic Factors

The current estimation is that approximately 400,000–500,000 septic episodes occur each year in the United States. These figures appear to be on the rise. Factors that are potentially responsible for the growing incidence of sepsis are listed in Table 8.9.

Pathophysiology

Sepsis and septic shock can be viewed as a constellation of signs and symptoms that are the body's response to infection, with cytokines (or substances triggered by them) being responsible for most of the manifestations. The cytokine cascade that can lead to sepsis begins with the interaction of bacterial endotoxin, a lipopolysaccharide (LPS) found on the surface membrane of gram-negative bacteria, and LPS-binding protein. LPS-binding protein binds the endotoxin molecule to receptors on CD14. This binding triggers activation of proinflammatory cytokines, such as tumor necrosis factor, interleukin-1, and interleukin-8, which in turn activate leukocyte–endothelial cell adhesion and clotting and trigger the release of vasodilatory factors. Bacterial superantigens bind directly to major histocompatibility molecules and CD4 cells, leading to massive activation of macrophages and T cells and encouraging the continued and

T ABLE 8.9. Potential factors in the increasing incidence of sepsis and septic shock

Greater awareness of and sensitivity for the diagnosis
More patients with compromised immune system (e.g., AIDS)
Increased use of cytotoxic and immunosuppressant agents
Malnutrition
Alcoholism
Malignancy
Diabetes mellitus
Greater number of transplant recipients and transplantation procedures
Increased use of aggressive invasive procedures in patient management and diagnosis
Greater number of resistant microorganisms
Greater number of elderly patients

excessive immune response that eventually leads to end-organ damage and shock.

Clinical Manifestations

The patient usually manifests symptoms and signs related to the primary focus of infection. However, patients may also manifest symptoms and signs related to other systems. Cutaneous signs are cyanosis and ischemic necrosis of peripheral tissue. Cellulitis, pustules, bullae, and hemorrhagic lesions may also be present. Gastrointestinal manifestations include nausea, vomiting, diarrhea, ileus, gastric ulceration with bleeding, and cholestatic jaundice.

Laboratory Findings

Neutrophilia or neutropenia, often accompanied by increased numbers of immature forms of polymorphonuclear leukocytes, is the most common laboratory abnormality in patients with sepsis. Thrombocytopenia occurs in 50% of patients, and frank disseminated intravascular coagulation (DIC) occurs in 2%–3%. Urinalysis shows proteinuria. With septic shock, acute tubular necrosis may develop with oliguria, azotemia, and cellular granular casts. During the early phases of sepsis, respiratory alkalosis occurs and arterial blood gases reveal an elevated pH and decreased partial pressure of carbon dioxide (P_{CO_2}). In septic shock, a metabolic acidosis develops with elevated lactate levels. At least two blood cultures should be obtained from different vein puncture sites. An electrocardiogram often shows nonspecific ST-T wave abnormalities. Chest x-ray may reveal underlying pneumonia. Abnormalities in serum electrolytes can include an elevated anion gap with reduction of the bicarbonate concentration and metabolic acidosis. Liver function tests include modest hyperbilirubinemia and elevations of the transaminases. Most patients with diabetes have hyperglycemia.

Differential Diagnosis

The differential diagnosis of sepsis and septic shock includes cardiac and pulmonary disorders, as well as substance abuse (Table 8.10).

Treatment

Sepsis is a medical emergency that requires immediate treatment of the local infection site, hemodynamic and respiratory support, and elimination of the offending microorganism. Oxygen, sufficient to maintain arterial oxygen saturation in excess of 95%, should be provided by nasal cannula or by mask. If respiratory failure occurs, intubation with mechanical ventilation is necessary. Because many patients have a relative depletion of intravascular volume, 1–2 L of crystalloids should be given intravenously over 1–2 hours. If volume resuscitation fails to increase blood pressure, pressor agents (e.g., dopamine or dobutamine) should be given.

A broad-spectrum regimen with activity against gram-positive and gram-negative organisms should be started (Table 8.11). Generally, drugs should be administered intravenously at maximum recommended dosages. Many physicians favor using at least two effective antimicrobial agents when treating patients with neutropenia who have gram-negative pneumonia and a two-drug synergistic combination when treating patients with serious enterococcal infection. Anaerobes are likely pathogens in intraabdominal infections, aspiration pneumonia, and abscesses. Infection of an intravascular catheter suggests the presence of methicillin-resistant *Staphylococcus* and the need for vancomycin (Vancocin).

In up to one-third of patients, no organism or source will be identified. Such patients require a broad-spectrum regimen, such as vancomycin with gentamicin (Garamycin) and metronidazole (Flagyl, Protostat) or ceftazidime (Ceptaz, Fortaz) with gentamicin. Early antifungal therapy with amphotericin B (Amphocin, Fungizone) should be considered in neutropenic, immuno-

T ABLE 8.10. Differential diagnosis of sepsis and septic shock

Myocardial infarction
Pulmonary embolism
Drug overdose
Occult hemorrhage
Cardiac tamponade
Rupture of an aortic aneurysm
Aortic dissection

T ABLE 8.11. Empirical therapy for sepsis

Associated condition	Usual pathogen	Recommended therapy
Neonatal sepsis	Group B streptococci Escherichia coli Listeria	Ampicillin and third-generation cephalosporin
Chronic alcoholism	Oral anaerobes Klebsiella sp.	Third-generation cephalosporin, levofloxacin (Levaquin), meropenem (Merrem), or cefepime (Maxipime)
Intraabdominal sepsis	Escherichia coli and other Enterobacteriaceae Anaerobes Enterococci	Ampicillin/sulbactam, Imipenem (Primaxin), Ticarcillin/clavulanic acid (Timentin)
Postviral influenza	Staphylococcus aureus	Nafcillin (Unipen)
Neutropenia	Enterobacteriaceae Pseudomonas aeruginosa Staphylococcus aureus Staphylococcus epidermidis	Third-generation cephalosporin, aminoglycoside and vancomycin (Vancocin)
Catheter	Staphylococcus epidermidis	

suppressed patients and in those who have been unresponsive to antibacterial regimens.

Prognosis

The outcome in patients with gram-negative sepsis depends more on host factors than on the virulence of the causative organisms. A major determinant of mortality is the presence of underlying disease (e.g., acute leukemia). The overall mortality in patients with gram-negative sepsis is about 25%.

Prevention

Prevention offers the best opportunity to reduce morbidity and mortality associated with sepsis. Measures include reducing the number of invasive procedures, limiting the use and duration of indwelling catheters, reducing the incidence and duration of profound neutropenia, aggressively treating localized infection, and immunizing against specific pathogens.

REFERENCES

1. Tyler KL, Martin JB, eds. *Infectious diseases of the central nervous system*. Philadelphia: FA Davis, 1993.

2. American Academy of Pediatrics. Dexamethasone therapy for bacterial meningitis in infants and children. In: Peter G, ed. *1997 red book: report*

of the Committee on Infectious Diseases, 24th ed. Elk Grove Village, IL: American Academy of Pediatrics, 1997:620–622.

3. Miller LG, Choi C. Meningitis in older patients: how to diagnose and treat a deadly infection. *Geriatrics* 1997;52 (8):43–44.

4. Schuchat A, Robinson K, Wenger JD, et al. Bacterial meningitis in the United States in 1995. Active Surveillance Team. *N Engl J Med* 1997; 337:970–976.

5. Quagliarello VJ, Scheld WM. Treatment of bacterial meningitis. *N Engl J Med* 1997;336:708–716.

6. Rosenstein N, Levine O, Taylor JP, et al. Efficacy of meningococcal vaccine and barriers to vaccination. *JAMA* 1998;279:435–439.

7. Ashwal S. Neurological evaluation of the patient with acute bacterial meningitis. *Neurol Clin* 1995;13:549–577.

8. McIntyre PB, Berkey CS, King SM, et al. Dexamethasone as adjunctive therapy in bacterial meningitis. A meta-analysis of randomized clinical trials since 1988. *JAMA* 1997;278:925–931.

9. Schaad UB, Kaplan SL, McCracken GH Jr. Steroid therapy for bacterial meningitis. *Clin Infect Dis* 1995;20:685–690.

10. Bleck TP, Greenlee JE. Approach to the patient with suspected central nervous system infections. In: Mandell GE, Bennett JE, Dolen R, eds. *Principles and practices of infectious disease,* 5th ed. Philadelphia: Churchill Livingstone, 2000:950–958.

11. Opal SM. Sepsis. In: Dale DC, Federman DD, eds. *Scientific american medicine.* New York: Scientific American 1998:1–11.

12. Noskin GA, Phair JP. Approach to the patient with bacteremia and sepsis. In: Humes HD, ed. *Kelley's textbook of internal medicine.* Philadelphia: Lippincott Williams & Wilkins, 2000:1918–1925.

13. Balk RA. Septic shock: pathophysiology. *Curr Opin Anesthes* 1998;7: 136–140.

14. Bone RC, Fisher CJ Jr, Clemmer TP, et al. Sepsis syndrome: a valid clinical entity. *Crit Care Med* 1989;17:389–393.

15. Cunha BA. Mimics of sepsis. In: Cunha BA, ed. *Infectious diseases in critical care medicine.* New York: Marcel Dekker, 1998:57–66.

16. Bernard GR, Christman JW, Cunha BA. Current thinking on sepsis treatment. *Patient Care* 1999;33(51):78–92.

17. Bone RC, Balk RA, Cerra FB, et al. American College of Chest Physicians/ Society of Critical Care Medicine Consensus Conference: definitions for sepsis and organ failure and guidelines for the use of innovative therapies in sepsis. *Chest* 1992;101:1644–1655.

CHAPTER 9

Renal

Richard B. Birrer

Acute renal failure is a medical emergency that can be encountered by any physician. It is defined as an abrupt decline in renal function, regardless of cause, that is sometimes accompanied by oliguria (urine output < 400 mL/day) or anuria (< 100 mL/day). Acute renal failure always results in the retention of nitrogenous wastes as measured by elevated serum creatinine and blood urea nitrogen (BUN) levels. Because acute renal failure is often reversible, successful management depends on distinguishing among various prerenal, intrarenal, and postrenal causes. An organized and systematic approach is essential because of the multiple etiologic factors and the possible devastating complications.

CHIEF COMPLAINT

The following are signs and symptoms of acute renal failure:

- Inability to urinate
- Lassitude
- Weakness
- Fatigue
- Dizziness
- Thirst
- Fever
- Rash
- Sore throat
- Syncope
- Flank or abdominal pain
- Edema

PATHOPHYSIOLOGY

The three basic categories of acute renal failure are *prerenal, intrarenal,* and *postrenal* (Table 9.1) (1). *Prerenal* azotemia, the most common cause of oliguria, is defined as a rapidly reversible rise in the serum creatinine due to renal hypoperfusion. No parenchymal damage occurs. Nonsteroidal antiinflammatory drugs (NSAIDs) and angiotensin-converting enzyme (ACE) inhibitors interfere with renal autoregulatory mechanisms, causing prerenal acute renal failure in patients with only mild hypovolemia or congestive heart failure.

147

T ABLE 9.1. Causes of acute renal failure

Prerenal
Hypovolemia
    Intravascular
        Hemorrhage
        Third space
            Burns
                Peritonitis
            Traumatized tissue
                Diuretic abuse
            Pancreatitis
            Postoperative ileus
            Nephrotic syndrome
            Cirrhosis
    Extravascular
        Gastrointestinal losses
        Urinary diuresis
            Skin/sweat losses
            Inadequate fluid intake
Impaired cardiac function
    Congestive heart failure
    Valvular heart disease
    Myocardial infarction
    Acute pulmonary embolism
    Pulmonary hypertension
    Constrictive pericarditis
    Positive pressure mechanical ventilation
    Pericardial tamponade
Renal vascular (venous or arterial) obstruction (bilateral)
    Thrombosis
    Embolism
    Dissecting aortic aneurysm
Increased renal vascular resistance
    Hepatorenal syndrome
    Anesthesia
    Surgery
    α-Adrenergic agonists
    NSAIDs
    ACE inhibitors
    Cyclosporine
    Radiocontrast agents
Peripheral vasodilatation
    Antihypertensive medications

T ABLE 9.1. Continued

    Anaphylactic shock
    CNS-mediated hypotension
    Bacteremia
Intrarenal
Ischemic
    Major surgery
        Hypotension
    Cardiogenic, septic, or hypovolemic shock
Nephrotoxic acute tubular necrosis
    Antiinfectives (aminoglycosides, penicillins, tetracyclines, amphotericin [Amphocin])
    Radiocontrast agents
    Myoglobinuria (rhabdomyolysis from crush/compartment syndromes)
        Hemoglobinuria (transfusion reactions)
        Chemotherapeutic agents (cisplatinol, methotrexate)
        Heavy metals
        Solvents
        Pesticides and fungicides
        Immunosuppressive agents (cyclosporine [Sandimmune])
        NSAIDs
Tubulointerstitial disease
    Multiple myeloma
        Drugs
    Crystals
        Infections
        Allergic interstitial nephritis
Glomerulonephritis
    Immune complex—mediated
        Hypocomplementemic
        Membranoproliferative
            Cryoglobulinemia
            Postinfectious
        Lupus nephritis
        Subacute bacterial endocarditis
    Goodpasture's syndrome
        Serum sickness
        Hemolytic uremic syndrome
        Thrombotic thrombocytopenic purpura
    IgA nephropathy
    With vasculitis
        Polyarteritis
            Drugs
        Antiglomerular basement membrane disease

continued on next page

TABLE 9.1. Continued

───

     Wegener's granulomatosis
        Pauci-immune renal vasculitis
   Other vascular causes
     Trauma
        Pregnancy (eclampsia, preeclampsia, abruptio placentae, postpartum renal failure, abortion, and
           HELLP syndrome)
     Cholesterol embolization
     Thrombotic microangiopathy
        Malignant hypertension

Postrenal
   Urethral obstruction
   Bilateral obstruction of ureters
     Intraureteral
        Edema
        Stones
        Necrotizing papillitis (from analgesics, diabetes, and sickle cell disease)
           Blood clots
        Pyogenic debris
        Sulfonamide and uric acid crystals
        Acyclovir (Zovirax)
           Pigments (myoglobin, hemoglobin)
     Extraureteral
        Pregnancy
        Pelvic abscess
        Pelvic hematoma
        Periureteral fibrosis
        Accidental ureteral ligation during surgery
        Tumor: prostate, cervix, uterus, endometrium
        Ascites
   Bladder neck obstruction
     Benign prostatic hypertrophy
     Bladder infection
     Bladder carcinoma
     Functional (ganglionic blocking agents or neuropathy)

───

ACE, angiotensin-converting enzyme; CNS, central nervous system; HELLP, hemolysis, elevated liver enzymes, low platelet count; NSAIDs, nonsteroidal antiinflammatory drugs.

Damage to the renal tissue proper constitutes *intrarenal* acute renal failure. Fifty percent of the renal mass must be lost before the creatinine clearance is affected. Therefore, the causes of acute renal failure often affect the kidneys bilaterally. Causes include a variety of hypoperfusive states (e.g., shock, aortofemoral bypass), resulting in tissue ischemia and acute tubular necrosis or direct toxic damage to the nephron (aminoglycosides). Prolonged renal ischemia (most common), pigmenturia, and nephrotoxinemia individually or synergistically produce acute tubular necrosis, which is considered acute renal failure when it is not the result of primary glomerular, interstitial, or vascular disorders. Acute renal failure and acute tubular necrosis are synonymous in the clinical setting.

Pathogenically, the ischemia causes tubular epithelia to swell, sloughing into and obstructing the tubular lumen as casts, which allows back-leak of tubular fluid and contributes to a decline in the glomerular filtration rate (Fig. 9.1). Intense intrarenal vasoconstriction (more than 50% reduction)

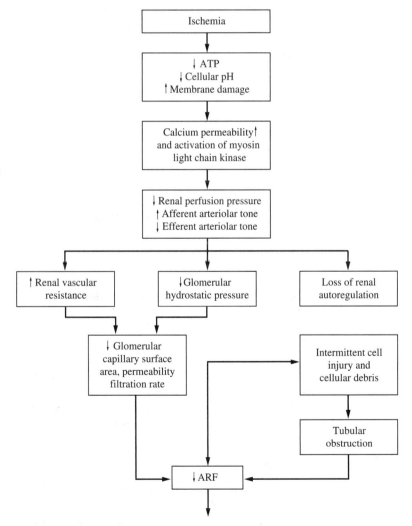

FIGURE 9.1. Pathogenesis of acute renal failure. ARF, acute renal failure.

completes the picture, although 50% of cases of postoperative acute tubular necrosis occur in the absence of documented hypotension. In a similar manner, necrosis and subsequent sloughing of tubular cells into the lumen, caused by medications, crystals, or pigments, can cause nephrotoxic acute tubular necrosis. Pathogenically, the renal blood flow and glomerular filtration rate are decreased due to ischemic insult and back-leak, leading to the vascular and tubular abnormalities that characterize acute renal failure. An increase in cellular calcium appears to be responsible.

Because the tissue half-life is more than 100 times the serum half-life, aminoglycoside-induced acute renal failure is dose-dependent and can occur even after cessation of administration (7–10 days after therapy is begun). Radiocontrast agents, whether administered intravenously, orally, or intraarterially, probably produce a post-hyperemic vasoconstriction via a calcium-dependent mechanism, although enhanced urate and oxalate excretion occur. The onset of acute renal failure is usually within 48 hours of administration, with peak serum creatinine levels occurring 3 to 5 days after the procedure. NSAIDs decrease prostaglandin synthesis by blocking cyclooxygenase, which leads to the depletion of vasodilatory eicosanoids, severe renal vasoconstriction, and reduced glomerular filtration rate, especially in the setting of comorbid states (cirrhosis, nephrotic syndrome, papillary necrosis). ACE inhibitors lower renal perfusion pressure and dilate the efferent arterioles by decreasing angiotensin II levels. Any condition that causes prerenal acute renal failure may cause intrarenal acute renal failure if the hypoperfusion is severe and prolonged (e.g., acute cortical necrosis).

Anuria suggests bilateral renal artery occlusion from atrial fibrillation, dissecting aortic aneurysm, or abdominal trauma. Acute renal vein thrombosis does not produce acute renal failure unless the thrombosis is bilateral. In adults, it is almost always secondary to preexisting nephrotic syndrome and glomerular disease or to an extension of an inferior vena cava thrombosis that involves the renal veins, as is seen in metastatic or local carcinoma or migratory thrombophlebitis. Acute renal failure develops in up to 30% of such cases.

Postrenal acute renal failure is relatively rare unless the obstruction is severe, prolonged, and bilateral. Irrespective of underlying cause, increased back-pressure on the renal tubules causes necrosis and sloughing and ultimately leads to a reduced glomerular filtration rate and renal blood flow (Fig. 9.1).

Any cause of oliguric failure may also cause nonoliguric failure; often the presence of oliguria reflects the severity, rather than the cause, of the disease.

CLINICAL MANIFESTATIONS

Acute renal failure may be asymptomatic and may be found serendipitously during the general evaluation and treatment of an unrelated disease state. Nonetheless, early indicators may be weight gain, oliguria, and edema.

In *prerenal* azotemia, the patient usually complains of thirst, sweating, nausea/vomiting, diarrhea, or dizziness in the upright position. He or she may have a history of overt fluid loss, diuretic use, or bleeding. The amount of dehydration is best assessed by serial weight checks. Collapsed neck veins, dry mucous membranes and axillas, decreased skin turgor, and orthostatic/postural changes in blood pressure and pulse may be noted. Distended neck veins, a third heart sound, and signs of pulmonary and peripheral edema suggest heart failure or volume overload.

A history of vasculitis; atrial fibrillation; chronic renal disease; diabetes; hypertension; use of intravenous drugs (usually illicit), antibiotics, or NSAIDs; sore throat or upper respiratory infection; a recent vascular catheterization; pigmenturia; or volume depletion are suggestive of an *intrarenal* cause of acute renal failure. Flank or back pain and/or abdominal pain is present in 30%-50% of cases. Symptoms of uremia are unusual, although nausea and vomiting are present in approximately 50% of cases. Fever is even more common and may be reflected in a raised white blood cell (WBC) count. A minority of patients with interstitial disease present with the classic triad of fever, rash, and arthralgia; eosinophilia in the blood and urine is characteristic. In general, the physical examination is of limited value in determining the cause of intrarenal acute renal failure but is of immense worth in assessing the severity of complications. New-onset hypertension may indicate glomerulonephritis. Careful inspection of the integument may provide other clues (e.g., purpura, cyanosis of a finger or toe tip, or livedo reticularis). Gross hematuria and the presence of the stigmata of systemic disease—for example, hematuria, hemoptysis, and rash in conditions such as lupus, Henoch-Schönlein purpura, and AIDS—are helpful. Acute cortical necrosis is characterized by anuria and signs of intravascular coagulation.

The diagnosis of *postrenal* renal failure is often apparent from the history and physical examination. Flank pain and tenderness are frequently present, although they are nonspecific. Renal colic classically occurs during the night or early morning hours (see Chapter 7). The onset is usually abrupt with crescendo pain that begins in the flank and extends laterally around the abdomen and into the groin. The pain, accompanied by nausea and vomiting, may radiate into the labia majora in women and into the testicles in men. A medical emergency is suggested by a history of fever and chills suggestive of a superimposed infection. The patient's skin is often pale, clammy, and cool. Tachycardia and hypertension may result from the agonizing pain. The abdominal examination is usually unremarkable except for a decrease in bowel sounds due to diminished peristalsis and costovertebral angle and flank tenderness, but even these findings are highly variable.

An abdominal mass (e.g., distended bladder [>500 mL], hydronephrotic kidney, or obstructing tumor) may be detected by palpation and percussion. Postoperative patients may leak urine through a wound. Edema from overhydration may be evident. Ileus is often present along with associated abdominal distention and vomiting. A rectal examination may identify an enlarged prostate. Patients who are at risk for endometrial carcinoma or endometriosis and who present with postrenal azotemia require a pelvic examination. Significant obstruction may be present without anuria or oliguria, despite acute renal failure. After an attempt at complete voiding, an estimation of the residual urine in the bladder should be made by straight catheter to evaluate the presence of urethral and bladder neck obstruction.

EPIDEMIOLOGIC FACTORS

The incidence of acute renal failure depends largely on the type of patient population. Approximately 1% of patients presenting to a hospital emergency department have acute renal failure. Etiologic factors include prerenal azotemia from a variety of causes (70%), obstructive uropathy (17%), and intrarenal pathologic processes (11%). One to five percent of all acute renal failure consists of glomerular, vascular, and interstitial disorders. Acute renal failure can affect 2%-5% of all patients in general medical and surgical wards; therefore, it is considered a disease of the hospitalized patient. Aminoglycoside nephrotoxicity develops in 5%-15% of patients treated with these drugs. Radiocontrast-induced acute renal failure occurs from 1.5% in a random population to 92% in individuals with an underlying disease (average 15%-25%). Thirty to sixty percent of patients with parenchymal acute renal failure do not have oliguria and may have outputs of more than 1,000 mL/day. This condition is called nonoliguric renal failure.

Obstruction of the urinary tract can occur at any age and can present as soon as urine production begins during the fourth month in utero (2). Hydronephrosis is present in 3.5%-3.8% of autopsies. The incidence of acute renal failure has increased in the elderly and in patients with complex illnesses, such as septicemia and multiorgan failure, whereas it has decreased in obstetric patients and in those undergoing elective surgery and hemodialysis.

Acute renal failure is associated with significant morbidity and a six- to eightfold increase in mortality. Although dialysis is available, 25% of patients with acute renal failure unassociated with trauma or surgery and 50%-70% of those with trauma-related acute renal failure die.

RISK FACTORS

Risk factors for acute tubular necrosis are as follows:

- Age > 60 years.
- Recent use of medications (NSAIDs, heavy metals, radiocontrast agents).
- Sepsis with prolonged hypotension.
- Myoglobinuria following trauma.
- Myocardial infarction.

- Dehydration.
- Diseases, such as myeloma, hyperuricemia, hypertension, peripheral vascular disease, diabetes mellitus, underlying renal insufficiency, cirrhosis with ascites, and refractory heart failure.

The most prevalent risk factors for NSAID-induced renal failure are as follows:

- Concurrent use of diuretics.
- Age >60 years.
- Comorbid states (e.g., nephrotic syndrome, atherosclerotic cardiovascular disease, renovascular disease, diabetes mellitus, acute gouty arthritis, cirrhosis, dysproteinurias, hypercalciuria, lupus nephritis, severe congestive heart failure, multiple myeloma).
- Large contrast load.
- Intravascular volume depletion.

The most prevalent risk factors for radiocontrast-induced renal failure are as follows:

- Acute liver failure.
- Age >55 years.
- Diabetes mellitus with neurovascular complications.
- Volume depletion.
- Recent nephrotoxic drug exposure.
- Proteinuria.
- Prior renal insufficiency.

The incidence and severity of acute renal failure following an intravenous pyelogram (IVP) rise with increasing levels of serum creatinine. Diabetic patients with normal renal function do not appear to be at risk for contrast-mediated nephropathy, but the risk rises significantly as the serum creatinine increases (50% with levels between 1.5 and 4.5 mg/dL and 90% with levels greater than 4.5 mg/dL).

DIAGNOSIS

The differential diagnoses of acute renal failure cover a wide range of organ system failure. These include all causes of altered mental status; sepsis; endocrinologic dysfunction of the adrenals, pancreas, and thyroid; heart failure; shock; and toxic syndromes.

Diagnosis of nonacute tubular necrosis intrarenal pathologic processes usually requires arteriography (recommended in cases of anuria), radionuclide renal scan, magnetic resonance imaging (MRI), and biopsy.

A supine abdominal radiograph provides presumptive evidence of kidney stones because 90% of them are radiopaque. The IVP establishes the diagnosis in nearly all cases of ureteral colic and demonstrates the severity of obstruction. Identification (cystoscopy and retrograde ureteral catheterization) and relief of obstruction, which may involve a minor (bladder catheterization) or major (ureteral stent or nephrostomy tube placement) surgical procedure, are the treatments for postrenal renal failure. Ultrasonography is the diagnostic test of choice and has a positive predictive value of 93%. Dilation of the urinary collecting system is detectable within 1–2 days of onset of obstruction. The percentage yield declines in the face of small shrunken kidneys and staghorn calculi. A retrograde pyeloureterogram should be ordered in cases of suspected obstruction whose ultrasonographic study is normal. Computed tomography (CT) is also useful. Because 90% of renal calculi are radiopaque, a KUB (kidney, ureter, bladder) flat plate of the abdomen should be ordered. In addition, small kidneys on KUB suggest advanced chronic renal pathology. The IVP shows characteristic poor visualization. A urine leak may be visible on a radionuclide renal scan; or, in cases of obstruction, retention of the isotope in the renal pelvis may be seen.

LABORATORY

The urine volume, sediment, and composition can be a clue to the cause of acute renal failure (Table 9.2). Accurate assessment may require bladder catheterization followed by hourly output measurements. About 50% of patients will be truly oliguric. In pre- and postrenal etiologies, the concentrating capacity of the kidney is preserved; and the routine urinalysis is typically normal. However, in postrenal partial obstructive etiologies, daily volumes may vary greatly and abolition of the renal concentrating ability may occur. In addition, 10% of renal lithiasis patients have gross hematuria; and 90% have positive findings on microscopy. Recovery from acute renal failure is characterized by a gradual increase, rather than a marked increase or decrease, from day to day. A complication should be suspected if the urine volume plateaus or decreases prematurely.

An active sediment with cellular debris, renal tubular epithelial cells, and tubular cell casts supports the diagnosis of acute renal failure. However, for the urine to contain only granular casts without tubular cell casts or renal tubule cells is not uncommon. The presence of a few white and red blood cells per high-power field and 1+ to 2+ proteinuria is compatible with the diagnosis of acute renal failure. Rarely, red blood cell (RBC) casts may be transiently noted. Large amounts of urinary protein and numerous RBC and WBC casts indicate acute renal failure from renal parenchymal disease. Pre- and postrenal azotemias are characterized by a lack of cellular elements and protein in the urine. Occasionally, severe congestive heart failure can produce urinary protein greater than 3 g/day in patients with prerenal acute renal failure. An abundance of crystals in the urine, such as urate or oxalate, suggests ethylene glycol or methoxyflorane toxicity. A urine dipstick that is positive for blood but negative for microscopic RBCs is suggestive of hemoglobinuria or myoglobinuria. The clinician should look for tissue, stones, or gravel and should have them analyzed.

TABLE 9.2. Urinary indices and composition in patients with acute renal failure

Location	Specific gravity	Sediment findings	U_{osm}	U/P_{osm}	Urine volume	BUN/creat.	RFI	FE_{Na}	U_{Na}	U/P_{urea}	U/P_{Cr}
Prerenal	>1.020	Normal; some hyaline/ granular casts	>500	>1.2	400–500	>20:1	<1	<1	<30	>20–30	>40
Intrarenal	<1.015	Brown granular casts; cellular debris	<400	<1.1	<400	<10:1	>2	>2	Variable	<20	<20
Postrenal	>1.020	Tubular cells and casts	Usually >350	<1.1	Variable	>20:1	>1	>1	Variable	Variable	<20

BUN/creat., ratio of blood urea nitrogen to creatinine; U_{osm} = urine osmolality; U/P_{osm}, U/P_{Cr}, U/P_{urea} = urine-to-plasma ratios of osmolality, creatinine, and urea, respectively; U_{Na} = urine sodium concentration (mEq/L); RFI = renal failure index* ($U_{Na}/U_{Cr}/P_{Cr}$); FE_{Na} = fractional sodium secretion.*

$$* = \left(\left[\frac{U_{Na} \times P_{CR}}{P_{Na} \times U_{CR}} \right] \times 100 \right)$$

day), hypocalcemia, hyperphosphatemia, hypermagnesemia, anemia, and platelet dysfunction.

REFERRAL

All patients with acute renal failure should be sent to the emergency department for immediate evaluation, treatment, and hospital admission. A urology consultation is appropriate in cases of postrenal acute renal failure. A nephrologist should be consulted for acute renal failure of unknown cause and for most cases of parenchymal acute renal failure.

MANAGEMENT

Emergency care consists of the following:

- Secure and protect the airway; provide oxygenation.
- Establish an IV line and provide fluid resuscitation if hypovolemia has occurred (watch for overload).
- Obtain an electrocardiogram and check for signs of hyperkalemia and incipient cardiac arrest.
- Implement frequent clinical monitoring of vital signs and inputs/outputs.

Careful balance of intake and output of fluid and electrolytes is extremely important in patients with both oliguric and nonoliguric acute renal failure (3,4). The management of the latter is more complex. If the daily urine volume is 500 mL or less and insensible losses are 500–750 mL, fluid restriction to less than 1 L per day is reasonable. However, daily urine and insensible losses in patients with nonoliguric failure may exceed 2 L/day. Daily measurements of weight and regular monitoring of vital signs are essential. Weight gain may reflect fluid retention from heart failure or from oliguria secondary to intrarenal acute renal failure; weight loss may indicate prerenal disease and volume depletion during the time period corresponding to a rise in serum creatinine. Periods of hypotension should be considered causative for prerenal disease or acute tubular necrosis.

Pre- and postrenal acute renal failures are usually immediately reversible. Prompt correction of the extracellular fluid volume and of the cause of cardiac failure or systemic vasodilatation (sepsis or excessive use of antihypertensive therapy) will improve the underlying prerenal azotemia and establish the diagnosis. In patients with normal baseline renal function, the reversal should take 1–2 days; recovery may be delayed in patients with substantial baseline renal impairment. Specifically, 300–500 mL of normal saline is administered; and the urine output is measured over the subsequent 1–3 hours. A favorable response is a urine volume increase of more than 50 mL/hour. The infusion should be continued to restore plasma volume and to correct dehydration because inadequate fluid management can lead to further renal hemodynamic deterioration, and eventual renal tubular ischemia

Thus, evaluation of urinary composition may be helpful in distinguishing the causes of acute renal failure. However, acute urinary tract obstruction for a few hours (postrenal acute renal failure) may be associated primarily with renal hypoperfusion and, thus, with a urinary composition similar to that seen in prerenal azotemia. In contrast, chronic urinary tract obstruction is associated with tubular dysfunction, and the urinary composition may resemble that of acute tubular necrosis.

A complete blood count (CBC) may demonstrate the thrombocytopenia and altered RBC morphology of hemolytic uremic syndrome. Complement is often decreased significantly in immune complex diseases. While liver enzyme functions may be elevated, a significant increase in lactic dehydrogenase (LDH) is a reliable indicator of renal infarction.

Interpret the serum creatinine level with caution because serious underlying renal disease may be present in the patient with a normal creatinine level. The patient's muscle mass must be considered when interpreting the level because a value of 1 mg/dL may represent considerable impairment in a small, asthenic individual. The Cockcroft-Gault formula can be used to correct the serum creatinine for a patient's body size, gender, and age (Fig. 9.2). Under normal circumstances, the serum creatinine increases 1-1.5 mg per dL per day in the complete absence of kidney function. Finally, the serum creatintine level may be falsely elevated without a true decrease in the glomerular filtration rate. Ketoacidosis caused by acetoacetate and the cephalosporin antibiotics interferes with the creatinine assay. Sulfa drugs and cimetidine (Tagamet) inhibit tubular secretion of creatinine.

The rise in BUN (10-20 mg per deciliter per day) may be more rapid than the increase in serum creatinine concentration (1-2 mg per deciliter per day) because the urea clearance in prerenal and postrenal etiologies is reduced. Thus, a BUN/creatinine ratio greater than 20:1 suggests a pre- or postrenal cause, whereas parenchymal disease is suggested by a BUN/creatinine ratio less than 10:1. However, the ratio may be falsely elevated with gastrointestinal hemorrhage, increased protein intake, or an elevated endogenous catabolic rate (e.g., fever, trauma). Alternatively, lower ratios (<20:1) may be seen in patients with liver disease, a lower catabolic rate, or a low-protein state. Furthermore, the serum creatinine reflects the glomerular filtration rate more accurately than does BUN. Therefore, the BUN/creatinine ratio should be interpreted with caution.

Other laboratory abnormalities to watch for are hyperkalemia (a rise of 0.3-0.5 mEq per L per day), reduced bicarbonate (a fall of 1-2 mEq per L per

---

Creatinine clearance = [140 − age (yr)] × body weight (kg)

72 × serum creatinine (mg/dL)

Note: Multiply the result by 0.85 if the patient is female.

FIGURE 9.2. Cockcroft Gault formula for determining creatinine clearance.

with fixed acute tubular necrosis. Discontinuance of antihypertensive drugs or diuretics can, by itself, cure apparent acute renal failure resulting from prerenal causes.

However, the rapidity of recovery from a *postrenal* condition depends on the completeness and duration of the obstruction. In nephrolithiasis, the most important factor relating to passage is the size of the stone. Approximately 90% of stones 4 mm or smaller that are located in the lower ureter will pass, whereas only 5%-10% of stones 8 mm or larger will do so. The most common sites at which stones are likely to be arrested are the narrowest portions of the ureter (the ureteropelvic junction, near the pelvic brim, or at the ureterovesical junction). Parenteral analgesia (50-100 mg meperidine [Demerol], 2-4 mg butorphanol [Stadol], or 10-15 mg morphine sulfate [Astramorph, Duramorph, Infumorph] intramuscularly) and ample hydration by mouth, if possible, are essential. Hospitalization is indicated if the stone is greater than 5-8 mm in diameter, if a high grade of ureteral obstruction exists, if pain or vomiting is intractable, if evidence of an infection is found, or if the patient has only one functioning kidney or has an underlying renal insufficiency. Note that profound diuresis (>1 L/hour) may follow the relief of a complete postrenal obstruction. Careful monitoring and aggressive fluid and electrolyte management prevent the complication of shock.

No known therapy exists for modifying the course of acute tubular necrosis; supportive measures to avoid complications are required (Table 9.3). Clinically, oliguria caused by a radiocontrast agent is usually abrupt, occurring within 24 hours of exposure, and is typically reversible; however, dialysis may occasionally be required to bridge the gap before normal renal function is restored.

In nonacute tubular necrosis of intrarenal origin, no increase in urine volume occurs following IV administration of a fluid challenge. The only current basis for diuretic use in acute renal failure is for management of volume status, not for hastening renal recovery or improved outcome. Furosemide (Lasix) may convert low urine output to high fixed output, but usually the rate of serum creatinine or the rise in BUN does not change. Following a fluid challenge, intakes and outputs must be carefully tracked in conjunction with BUN, creatinine, and electrolytes.

Regulation of protein and calorie intake is important for patients with acute renal failure. The development of azotemia in chronic renal failure can be slowed by dietary protein restriction (e.g., 30-50 g/day). To minimize the rate of endogenous catabolism, adequate nonprotein calories in the form of carbohydrates and essential amino acids should be added.

Complications must be identified early and managed aggressively (5,6). Although intermittent dialysis is frequently needed to avoid the symptoms of uremia and the unresponsive complications of acute renal failure, no evidence shows that dialysis shortens the course of acute renal failure. Indeed, serious complications (e.g., hypotension and arrhythmias) and delayed renal function recovery may follow the initiation of dialysis.

T ABLE 3.1.   Complications of acute renal failure

Metabolic
  Hyperuricemia
  Hyperkalemia
  Hyponatremia
  Hypocalcemia, hyperphosphatemia
  Metabolic acidosis
  Hypermagnesemia
Neurologic
  Seizures
  Somnolence[a]
  Coma[a]
  Asterixis
  Neuromuscular irritability
Infectious
  Sepsis
  Pneumonia
  Urinary tract infection
  Wound infection
Gastrointestinal
  Nausea[a]
  Vomiting[a]
Cardiopulmonary
  Pericarditis[a]
  Arrhythmias
  Hypertension
  Pleuritis[a]
  Congestive heart failure
  Pulmonary edema
Hematologic
  Hemorrhagic diathesis[a]
  Coagulopathies
  Anemia[a]
Miscellaneous
  Volume overload
    Nitrogenous fetor[a]
  Serositis[a]

[a]Uremic syndrome.

PROGNOSIS/FOLLOW-UP

The prognosis of acute renal failure depends on the patient's overall health, the severity and cause of the disease, and the number and type of complications. Overall, the prognosis is poor, with mortality ranging from 20% to 85%, and parallels the rise of serum creatinine. The average mortality rate is 50% (50% infection, 20% congestive heart failure, 10% gastrointestinal bleeding, 10% hyperkalemia, and 10% respiratory failure). Acute renal failure in the intensive care setting (associated with burns, severe trauma, and multiple clinical complications) has a 75% mortality rate, most commonly due to sepsis from urinary or pulmonary sites. Therefore, urinary catheters should be removed as soon as possible. Drug-induced acute renal failure is usually mild and is generally reversible. The prognosis for patients with nonoliguric renal failure is better (5%–32% mortality) than for those with oliguric renal failure (50% mortality).

Prerenal and postrenal acute renal failures are frequently reversible. Acute cortical necrosis has a poorer prognosis than acute tubular necrosis. Advanced age, repeated episodes of acute tubular necrosis, hypercatabolic metabolism, multiple complications, intensive care setting, and serious underlying disease are all associated with higher morbidity and mortality rates for acute tubular necrosis. The mortality rate rises 30% for each organ system that fails. For example, the rate rises eightfold when respiratory failure occurs with renal failure; hypercatabolic states double the mortality rate, liver failure triples it, and heart disease triples or quadruples it. By comparison, acute tubular necrosis that follows obstetric complications, rhabdomyolysis, or nephrotoxicity is associated with a better prognosis.

Patients who undergo dialysis are at highest risk for death. The mortality rate for primary kidney disease is 25%; for those who have major cardiovascular or gastrointestinal surgery, the rate is 75%–80%; and for those with severe burns, it is greater than 90%. For patients who survive acute renal failure, the prognosis is generally good. Of the 50% of patients who survive acute renal failure, 15% have a complete recovery; 25% have an incomplete recovery but stable renal functions; and 5%–30% have an incomplete recovery and slowly progress to end-stage renal disease.

PATIENT EDUCATION/PREVENTION

Identification of high-risk patients and tailored therapy for other disorders can prevent acute renal failure by attenuating kidney insult (6). In patients with documented renal compromise, daily body weight checks are warranted, as is restriction of magnesium, potassium, and dietary sodium intake. NSAIDs and ACE inhibitors should be used with caution in patients suffering from or predisposed to congestive heart failure or hypotension. The smallest effective dosages should be used for the shortest possible time. Renal function should be carefully monitored, and the drugs should be discontinued immediately if progressive renal dysfunction becomes evident. The administration of IV saline prior to a contrast study can significantly reduce the risk of nephrotoxicity in high-risk patients (from 70% to 22% in those with renal insufficiency, from 61% to 18% in those without diabetes, and from 92% to 33% in those with diabetes). Diuretics are not helpful. Hydration and salt loading are also essential for patients receiving amphotericin or cisplatin and for patients who are in the postoperative stage.

If nausea develops with vomiting, pain becomes intractable, or fever and chills occur in association with a kidney stone, the patient should return to care. Even after the stone has been passed, a urologic workup is necessary.

CONCLUSION

Acute renal failure consists of a wide variety of diagnostically and therapeutically challenging renal diseases, most of which are drug induced. Acute renal failure is a common problem that is not restricted to critical care areas. Many iatrogenic factors are predictable, preventable, and reversible. Once acute renal failure has occurred, treatment options are limited and await an improved understanding of the pathophysiologic processes of this diverse disorder.

REFERENCES

1. Brady HR, Brenner BM, Lieberthal WE. Acute renal failure. In: Brenner BM, ed. *The kidney*, 5th ed. Philadelphia: WB Saunders, 1996:48–87.

2. Martinez-Maldonado M, Kumjian DA. Acute renal failure due to urinary tract obstruction. *Med Clin N Am* 1990;74:919–932.

3. Edelstein CL, Ling H, Wangsiripaisan A, Schrier RW. Emerging therapies for acute renal failure. *Am J Kidney Dis* 1997;30(5 Suppl 4):S89–S95.

4. Biology of acute renal failure: therapeutic implications. *Kidney Int* 1997; 52(4):1102–1115.

5. Mehta R. Therapeutic alternatives to renal replacement for critically ill patients in acute renal failure. *Semin Nephrol* 1994;14:64–82.

6. Anderson RJ. Prevention and management of acute renal failure. *Hospital Pract (Off Ed)* 1993;33(8):61–75.

CHAPTER 10

. . . .

Allergic

Vicken Y. Totten and Fitzgerald Alcindor

Acute allergic emergencies in the office are those that may become life-threatening within 30 minutes or less if not treated. The most important diagnostic tool is a clinical suspicion of an acute allergic or allergic-like reaction. The diagnosis is confirmed by physical examination. Respiratory emergencies of all sorts are among the most common life-threatening problems encountered in clinical practice. They must be recognized and treated promptly. (1)

Medications needed to treat the allergic or pseudo-allergic reaction include oxygen, normal saline, epinephrine, and steroids. Equipment for administering medications intravenously, syringes, and nebulizers complete the list of essential equipment. Antihistamines are reserved for subsequent treatment. These medications prevent the degranulation of mast cells and block the allergic cascade initiated by histamine; by the time that the patient has a life-threatening reaction, the opportunity to prevent degranulation has passed.

This chapter covers the recognition and office treatment of anaphylaxis, anaphylactoid reactions, and angioneurotic edema. These conditions are contrasted with large and small local reactions to hymenopteran envenomation. Latex allergy is treated separately. Anaphylaxis differs from anaphylactoid reactions primarily by mechanisms at the cellular level; as the initial treatment is the same, the difference between the states will not be belabored.

Asthma, though it may be partially allergically mediated, is covered in Chapter 3 and will not be discussed here. Angioedema, which may not be allergic in nature, will be covered in this chapter because it can produce life-threatening swelling.

ANAPHYLAXIS AND ANAPHYLACTOID REACTIONS

Chief Complaint

A 12-year-old boy is undergoing intravenous pyelography in radiology down the hall from your office when the radiologist calls to ask you if you have any diphenhydramine (Benadryl, Banophen) and oxygen. He thinks the patient is having an allergic reaction.

Clinical Manifestations

The boy is recumbent, alert, in moderate respiratory distress, and wheezing. He is bright red all over and is scratching at his chest. On physical examination, he has a blood pressure of 70/50 mm Hg and a heart rate of 130 beats per minute and is breathing rapidly. He seems anxious but cooperative.

Epidemiologic Factors

The current estimation is that 1%–2% of patients who receive radiopaque contrast media have anaphylactoid reactions (2,3). Fortunately, deaths from allergic reactions are rare in the United States.

However, allergic reactions are not limited to radiopaque contrast media. Almost any parenteral injection can trigger anaphylactic shock, even injections of steroids (4). Antibiotics, foreign proteins (e.g., horse serum or animal-based insulins), and egg-based vaccinations account for the majority of anaphylactic reactions caused by therapeutic agents. More common triggers of anaphylactic or anaphylactoid reactions are nonmedicinal ingestants or inhalants. Foods frequently implicated include tree nuts or legumes (4), eggs, seafood, or preparations containing herbs or pollen. The variable presence of food preservatives, such as sodium and potassium bisulfites, may explain inconsistent food reactions. Endogenous triggers include hormones, such as progesterone, and exercise. Finally, latex can precipitate anaphylaxis. Latex is found in such a wide variety of products that an ever-increasing segment of the population has been sensitized.

The propensity to severe allergic reactions is rarely outgrown, and allergies appear to be increasing in prevalence. Food allergies often manifest early in life, frequently during the first known exposure. They may be life-threatening and may require emergency management. Accidental ingestions are common, frequently occur outside of the home, and often require emergency treatment. For this reason, persons at high risk for anaphylaxis are advised to carry epinephrine for initial management of an acute reaction.

Risk Factors

Persons with a family or personal history of other allergic reactions, previous anaphylactic reactions to other substances, or atopy are at particular risk. In one study, atopy was present in 54% of patients who developed anaphylaxis (5). Although the fact that one does not react to a substance on first encounter is a truism, clinically a reaction may appear to have occurred on first exposure if the actual first exposure was temporally remote or clinically unapparent.

Pathophysiology

Anaphylaxis is an immediate, life-threatening, general allergic reaction mediated by a variety of substances. The final common pathways result in vasodilatation and increased capillary permeability, which in turn causes a distributive shock and may cause mechanical blockage of end bronchioles, small vessels, or the gastrointestinal (GI) tract. The initial bioactive substances released by mast cells activate H_1 and H_2 receptors. Eosinophil-releasing factors then cause release of secondary enzymatic mediators of neutrophil chemotactic activity (NCA). These enzymes are released into the general circulation, last for 10–20 hours, and account for the second peak and the late-phase asthmatic responses (6).

Diagnosis

The diagnosis of a full-blown anaphylactic reaction is not difficult. Symptoms include massive generalized vasodilatation, causing a high-outflow type of shock and, potentially, cardiovascular collapse. Pruritus is almost universal. The vasodilatation may manifest as diffuse cutaneous urticaria but may also precipitate a variety of GI symptoms caused by gut wall edema, such as sensations of fullness, vomiting, diarrhea, abdominal cramps, and bowel obstruction. In the airway, diffuse edema coupled with acute bronchospasm may result in airway obstruction and even in death (7).

When anaphylaxis presents in a form fruste (incomplete manifestation), the differential diagnoses include angioedema (which is not associated with pruritus); various cutaneous allergic reactions, including isolated urticaria (which does not include airway symptoms), shock from any other cause (rarely vasodilatory; most forms of shock are associated with pallor); asthma (with a history of previous wheezing episodes); or pulmonary edema (which presents with hypertension and frothy sputum; see Chapter 3).

Airway obstructions that may mimic anaphylaxis include epiglottitis (with severe sore throat and fever, muffled voice, and tripod position), supraglottitis (again with systemic illness), retropharyngeal or peritonsillar abscess (which can often be felt or seen in the retropharynx), laryngospasms, foreign body aspiration, tumor, factitious anaphylaxis, or globus hystericus. In difficult cases, laryngoscopy (either direct or indirect) may help distinguish the edema of anaphylaxis from the normal vocal cords seen with the above causes of respiratory distress.

Diagnostic Tests

Diagnostic tests beyond the physical examination are not indicated; immediate treatment is lifesaving. In the future, mast cell tryptase may prove to be a definitive marker (8).

Management

Medications

- Oxygen—can be safely administered at any flow rate needed to maintain oxygenation but is only a temporizing measure.
- Epinephrine (adrenalin)—first-line treatment. Can be given as 0.01 mL/kg of 1:1,000 solution subcutaneously or as 1 mg of either 1:1,000 or 1:10,000 solution by nebulization. Either route should be safe in an office

setting; paramedics may also give epinephrine via an endotracheal tube or, possibly, by an intravenous line in the most critical cases.

- Methylprednisolone or other steroids (Medrol, Solu-Medrol)—may be helpful at terminating the acute episode and halting the inflammatory cascade. May be safely given intravenously, intramuscularly, or orally.
- Beta agonists (albuterol [Proventil, Ventolin, Airet])—administered by nebulization in an acute situation; beta agonists reverse potentially lethal bronchospasm.
- Theophylline (Aquaphyllin, Elixomin)—although it is a weak beta agonist, it is rarely useful in an acute episode of anaphylaxis and is not approved for this use by the U.S. Food and Drug Administration.
- Atropine—can be administered subcutaneously, intramuscularly, or intravenously in doses ranging from 0.005 to 0.01 mg/kg to reduce bronchospasm and GI reactivity. An off-label method of administration, occasionally used in the emergency department but safe for use in an office, is to nebulize up to 1 mg of the intravenous solution.
- Diphenhydramine—helps to prevent late progression of the allergic cascade but is not effective in terminating the initial episode. Can be given orally, intramuscularly, or intravenously.
- H_2 blockers, such as cimetidine (Tagamet)—function as nonsedating antihistamines to prevent recurrence or late progression, although this is an off-label use of this drug.

Initial management for all anaphylactic reactions is administration of epinephrine. The dose is 0.01 mg/kg or, for an adult, from 0.3 mL of 1:1,000 solution subcutaneously to 1.0 mg of 1:10,000 solution intravenously every 5 minutes. Epinephrine should be administered with caution to the elderly or those with cardiovascular disease.

Local measures may slow absorption of the inciting agent. Local measures are, in part, dependent on the site of the contact; but for stings or intramuscular injections, locally applied ice, tourniquets, or a local infiltration of epinephrine may be indicated.

If laryngeal edema predominates, epinephrine can be given by nebulization: either 10 mL of the 1:10,000 solution directly in the nebulizer chamber or 1 mL of 1:1,000 solution diluted with 9 mL of saline. Persistent bronchospasm may be improved by inhaled beta agonists or by nebulized epinephrine. The H_2 blockers seem to add to the effectiveness of diphenhydramine in reducing urticaria and in blocking the effects of histamine release. They are also nonsedating.

Referral

Referral may be indicated for allergen testing, which should only be done in a controlled environment with resuscitation capabilities. After allergen testing, desensitization may be indicated because avoidance of the offending agent, though always prudent, is not always possible.

Follow-up

If the symptoms of anaphylaxis have been mild and if the patient has responded, observation in the office or emergency department for several hours followed by discharge with continued use of steroids, conventional antihistamines, and possibly H_2 blockers is sufficient. Patients with moderate or severe reactions should be monitored in the hospital for 24–48 hours because of the risk of delayed return of symptoms.

Patient Education

Any patient who has suffered an anaphylactic reaction should be taught to avoid the inciting agent completely by carefully reading labels and understanding related agents. Patients should be instructed to seek medical treatment immediately after an exposure, even if they have self-treated and believe that they have responded. Furthermore, patients should carry a kit for self-administration of epinephrine (EpiPen, AnaKit) and should be instructed on how and when to use it. The patient's friends and relatives should also be taught how to use the kit. Caution the patient that the kit deteriorates quickly in the glove compartment of a car because of the intense summer heat and that it should be replaced every 2 years, even if not used.

ANGIOEDEMA

Chief Complaint

"My lips are swollen." A 48-year-old African-American woman presents to the office because she woke up this morning with a tight feeling in her lips. Her husband noticed that her lips seemed swollen. She is generally healthy except for hypertension, for which she takes enalapril (Vasotec) 5 mg/day. She has no known allergies, has not eaten any unusual foods, and has never had an episode like this; no one else in the family is sick or affected. She denies any recent bites or stings.

Clinical Manifestations

Her lips are at least twice their normal size and are asymmetrically swollen with more involvement of the left side of her face and the left side of her tongue. Her speech is somewhat muffled from the swelling of her tongue. Vital signs (including blood pressure) are normal, and her lungs are clear.

Epidemiologic Factors

Angioedema is a nonpruritic, localized, and generally well-demarcated non-pitting edema of deep subcutaneous tissues. It predominantly affects the head and intraoral areas. The mechanism is unclear. The incidence is higher in persons of African descent than in those of European descent.

The incidence of acute angiotensin-converting enzyme (ACE) inhibitor-induced angioedema is low (0.1%-0.2% of users) but can be considered a potentially life-threatening adverse effect of ACE inhibitor therapy (9). It rarely, if ever, starts with the first dose of an ACE inhibitor. Rather, after years of uneventful hypertension control, the patient manifests facial edema of sudden onset. The risk to life is from mechanical obstruction of the airway. ACE inhibitor–induced angioedema rarely extends below the glottis but can occasionally involve the larynx.

Even rarer than ACE inhibitor-induced angioedema is hereditary angioedema (HAE). HAE is recurrent. It is caused by an autosomally dominant C_1 esterase inhibitor deficiency (10). HAE primarily affects the airway, face, and extremities; but it can also present with (sometimes solely) GI symptoms, such as recurrent bouts of abdominal pain with nausea, vomiting, or diarrhea, when the intestinal mucosa is involved (11). Trauma and stress may be precipitating factors. Symptoms typically last 48-72 hours, but they can last from a period of 4 hours up to a week. Treatment includes prophylactic therapy with attenuated androgens or antifibrinolytic agents (12). Treatment is fresh frozen plasma (FFP) with a C_1 inhibitor. As in ACE inhibitor-induced angioedema, neither epinephrine nor steroid administration is useful. Danazol (Danocrine) may be used for long-term prophylaxis (13).

Risk Factors

The risk factors for angioedema include the following:

- African descent.
- Therapy with ACE inhibitors.
- Therapy with angiotensin II receptor antagonist (14).
- Family history of angioedema.

Pathophysiology

Angioedema differs from urticaria in that reactions are not confined to the dermis. Stimulation of H_1 and H_2 receptors causes release of mediators of inflammation, especially prostaglandins, leukotrienes, and kinins. Small blood vessels dilate, and their walls become permeable to fluids and proteins. Unlike anaphylaxis, angioedema tends to be restricted to a contiguous area, which typically is systemic.

IgE is the most common trigger for histamine release in urticaria; however, angioedema can also be triggered by cold, exercise, various drugs, and local trauma. A great deal of controversy about the appropriate therapy exists. On a theoretical basis, both H_1 and H_2 blockers should attenuate the physiologic response, but clinically neither seems particularly effective. Antileukotrienes should block a portion of the inflammatory cascade but, to date, have not been tested in angioedema.

Differential Diagnosis

- Urticaria—raised salmon-colored area of local, superficial skin edema. Also known as "welts."
- Local injury or trauma.
- Insect envenomation—a sting or fang mark can often be found.
- Anaphylaxis—see above.

Management

Generally, the treatment of ACE inhibitor-induced angioedema is not medical. The literature does not support the effectiveness of epinephrine. Steroids are only of modest benefit, and antihistamines are not effective (9,13). Leukotriene inhibitors are not approved by the U. S. Food and Drug Administration (FDA) for treatment of either type of angioedema but may be safe.

Treatment is primarily supportive. Administer oxygen and observe closely. The initial severity and speed of progression or remission will determine whether the patient should be observed in the office or the hospital. Since reactions typically diminish over 12 to 24 hours, referral to an emergency department may be more prudent, unless the patient presents early to the office. The ACE inhibitor should be withdrawn and should not be restarted. Mechanical obstruction of the airway is the prime threat to life. If swelling involves the pharynx or tongue, consider early intubation with a standby operative airway (cricothyrotomy or tracheostomy).

Referral

When the patient is taking an ACE inhibitor and can be adequately managed without this class of drugs, one may assume that withdrawing the ACE inhibitor will suffice. A person who develops acute angioedema without ACE inhibitors will need referral to an immunologist to determine if he or she has hereditary angioedema.

Follow-up

The disease course usually resolves within five days (often within 24 hours). Subsequently, the patient's hypertension or renal disease should not be managed with ACE inhibitors since the angioedema can recur.

Patient Education

The patient should be counseled to avoid ACE inhibitors in the future. If there is suspicion of hereditary angioedema, the patient should be referred to an immunologist for confirmation of the diagnosis and advice in management.

ENVENOMATIONS AND STINGS

Chief Complaint

A woman brings her 8-year-old son to the office because he was stung on the hand by a bee, and now his whole arm is swollen. She is sure he is allergic and wants him to get an "allergy shot."

Clinical Manifestations

The child is alert and has normal vital signs. A blanched mark is found over the first metacarpal, and fiery red edema extends to the biceps. Some patchy erythema is discovered over the upper arm, but no lesions are seen on other body parts. The axillary nodes are not enlarged, and the lungs are clear.

Epidemiologic Factors

Hymenopteran envenomation is caused by the sting (not the bite) of any member of the order Hymenoptera, which includes bees and wasps. Ants are closely related; although ants usually attack by biting, some ants do sting. Ant stings may cross-react with hymenopteran stings. Envenomation can produce either local or systemic reactions. Local reactions, no matter how large, are not considered allergic and do not require desensitization therapy. They are not a threat to life unless they involve the airway. Local reactions are essentially contiguous, although at their edges they may be patchy. Systemic reactions, on the other hand, are usually allergic in nature and can be life-threatening. Allergic reactions can include anaphylaxis (see above).

Risk Factors

- Previous large local reactions to insect venom.
- Family history of allergies.
- Factors that attract insects.

Bees are vegetarian and are attracted to flowers, bright clothing, and sweet scents. Hornets, yellow jackets, and wasps are carnivorous. They are attracted to meat or carrion and therefore may congregate near garbage cans. All hymenopterans need water, and some use mud as a building material. Many may congregate near muddy places in the summer.

Pathophysiology

Venoms differ somewhat among bees, yellow jackets, hornets, and wasps. All contain hyaluronidase and various phospholipases that spread the venom. Yellow jacket venom also contains kinins, whereas hornet venom includes acetylcholine. All persons react to these vasoactive poisons with local redness and pain (at least), depending on the dose injected.

Diagnosis

Differential Diagnosis

Other diagnoses to be considered include the following:
- Other insect bites—spider bites tend to be painless initially and later necrose; mosquito bites typically itch but have less erythema than hymenopteran bites.
- Local trauma.
- Urticaria.
- Angioedema.

Stings by honeybees rarely become infected, whereas stings from the carnivorous hymenopterans become infected more frequently. The only hymenopteran that loses its stinger in the wound is the honeybee. Since the avulsed stinger remains attached to the venom sacs, it may continue to inject venom for several minutes after the bee has fled. Fire ant stings frequently form a sterile pustule within 24 hours; the pustule is considered diagnostic for this insect's venom.

Management

Generally, medications, except for comfort, are not needed. However, if concerned about a severe reaction or the potential for anaphylaxis, treat as if for anaphylaxis (see "Anaphylaxis and Anaphylactoid Reactions" above).

Initial management of any envenomation is to prevent further venom from entering the body. Since honeybees lose their venom sac along with their stinger, the sac may continue to pulsate and may inject more venom for several minutes. A retained stinger should not be grasped with fingers or forceps, as this only compresses the sac further. Rather, a thin flat object should be scraped along the skin surface in hopes of catching one of the barbs and pulling the stinger out without further injection of venom. Fingernails, credit cards, and butter knives are suitable objects.

Local cooling minimizes the spread of venom and may decrease edema and itching. Antihistamines may decrease some of the redness and itching. The sedative actions of the first-generation antihistamines can help the patient endure the sting; nonsedating antihistamines may be less effective. Meat tenderizers that contain papaverine may denature the venom.

When an allergic component is manifested by urticaria, epinephrine, 0.005-0.01 mg/kg (usually 0.3 mg of 1:1,000 solution in an adult), provides almost immediate relief of itching but does not last more than 30-60 minutes. Steroids, either topically or orally, can be used to decrease the itching; 5 mg of prednisone daily for 3-5 days is recommended. Minor analgesics may be of benefit. The only potential long-term therapy is desensitization.

Most persons are stung only once or a few times. Commercial honey workers, agricultural workers, and particularly unlucky persons may suffer many stings. The volume of poison injected can cause shock and death, even in a person who is not allergic. Such persons should be managed in the emergency department or another intensive care setting. The primary treatment for massive envenomation is supportive therapy, with attention to airway, fluid resuscitation, and pump failure. Hymenopteran antivenoms are available and should be used early. Advice for managing a massive envenomation may be available from your local poison control center or a local agricultural college. Identifying the species of insect may be helpful.

Referral

Referral to an allergist for desensitization is prudent if a patient has had a potentially life-threatening reaction. In addition, the patient should be counseled on ways of avoiding additional stings. The patient should go to the emergency department if any evidence of shock or potential for airway compromise is found (anaphylaxis or large local reaction involving airway, mouth, lips, and tongue).

Follow-up

In most cases, the reaction to a sting vanishes in a few days and requires no medical monitoring. Large local reactions, involving the head or face, or an entire limb or equivalent body area should be monitored daily for spread to airways or other vital structures. Very rarely, the sting site will necrose, forming an eschar.

Patient Education

Anyone who has had an envenomation is potentially at risk for anaphylaxis. The most important education is how to avoid attracting hymenopterans, many of which are meat eaters. Honeybee-reactive persons should avoid bright clothing and flowery scents. Any allergic person should wear light-colored, protective clothing and should avoid areas that specifically attract the more aggressive yellow jackets (trash cans, picnic areas, and muddy water holes).

The patient who has had a severe reaction should also be instructed on the use of a commercial kit containing epinephrine and should carry it whenever he or she may be at risk of stings. Family members and friends should also be instructed on use of the kit. The patient should be counseled that the kit is only a temporizing measure while seeking medical help.

LATEX ALLERGIES

Chief Complaint

One of your patients is a 42-year-old nurse at the local hospital's emergency department. She is scheduled for a pelvic examination. After taking a Pap smear, you do a bimanual exam. A few moments after the examination, she complains of sudden vaginal itching, nausea, respiratory distress, and a sense of her throat closing. She also says that she experienced itching and dryness of her hands for years when using powdered latex gloves, so she switched to vinyl gloves; but she has never really considered herself to be allergic to latex.

Clinical Manifestations

The respiratory rate is 24/min, and the heart rate is 110 beats per minute. The rest of her vital signs are stable. She is anxious. Her lips are swollen, but her tongue and pharynx appear normal. She has mild wheezing. A call goes to 911; and, while waiting for the ambulance, you administer 0.3 mL of a 1:1,000 epinephrine solution subcutaneously. Then you give 50 mg of diphenhydramine and 40 mg of prednisolone orally. She seems better when the medics arrive and administer oxygen. Later, from a call to the emergency department, you learn that she improved and was discharged after 6 hours of observation.

Epidemiologic Factors

Latex is ubiquitous in modern society. It is used in the health care and food preparation industries to prevent transmission of microorganisms, especially HIV and other blood-borne diseases (15). Mechanics, painters, domestic workers, and homemakers may use latex or vinyl gloves to protect their hands from dirt or chemicals. Latex condoms are touted as the only pregnancy- and disease-preventing prophylactic.

Natural latex has a unique combination of strength, flexibility, and elasticity that makes it the material of choice for a variety of medical products, including examination gloves. Unfortunately, routine use of latex in the health care setting may be detrimental to patients and caregivers with a history of natural rubber latex hypersensitivity reactions (15).

Approximately 50% of health care workers have developed asthma, rhinorrhea, conjunctivitis, and secondary sinusitis attributable to type I reactions to latex. Of these, about 10% are at risk for anaphylaxis (16). Persons with spina bifida, others who undergo multiple surgical procedures, latex industry workers, housekeepers, food handlers, and individuals with food allergies to plant products that carry allergens cross-reactive to latex (such as banana, kiwi, avocado, and chestnuts) are at increased risk of anaphylaxis (17). Ten percent of people with spina bifida have overt allergy, and 50–60% have been found to have IgE antibodies specific to latex. In England, 3% of the population has latex sensitivity (18).

Risk Factors

The following are known risk factors for latex allergies:

- Exposure to latex.
- Known allergy to related compounds: banana, kiwi, avocado, and chestnuts.

Natural latex from the rubber tree *Hevea brasiliensis* is a potent allergen. The most important risk factor is repeated exposure. Since the onset of the AIDS epidemic in the 1980s and the subsequent institution of universal (standard) precautions and the increased use of condoms, the number of persons coming into contact with latex rubber has skyrocketed (19). Even police officers and firefighters now use gloves in medical encounters. Health care and rubber industry workers, children with spina bifida, or others undergoing repeated surgeries early in life are at special risk (20). Up to 36% of persons with atopia or a history of delayed-type hypersensitivity will develop latex allergy (21). How much of the current increase in latex allergy is attributable to the replacement of talc with cornstarch as glove donning powder is unclear. Cornstarch is more easily air-borne than talc and has been implicated in an increase in occupational asthma. The change in powder has also coincided with the rapid increase in latex glove allergy (22).

Pathophysiology

Type I or immediate hypersensitivity is mediated by IgE and IgG_4 and is the underlying cause of anaphylaxis in most cases (10). The binding of an allergen to IgE leads mast cells and basophils to release cellular mediators, such as histamine and platelet-activating factor, that initiate the inflammatory cascade that can present clinically as anaphylaxis.

Type II reactions, also called cytotoxic reactions, occur when circulating IgG or IgM binds to a cell-bound antigen. An example is the red cell lysis of transfusion reactions.

Type III reactions involve the formation of antigen–antibody complexes (immune complexes) that get deposited on specific organs or tissues and cause damage if not cleared by the reticuloendothelial system. The complex activates complement in preparation for phagocytosis. Classic examples are serum sickness and poststreptococcal glomerulonephritis.

Type IV (delayed hypersensitivity) is a cell-mediated reaction whereby sensitized T lymphocytes and macrophages initiate the inflammatory process in 48–72 hours. No antibody is involved. Delayed hypersensitivity plays no role in the pathogenesis of anaphylaxis. Examples include tuberculosis; leprosy; chlamydial infections; lymphogranuloma venereum; helminthic infections, such as schistosomiasis; and hypersensitivity pneumonitis (23).

Discussion

Natural rubber latex can cause immediate hypersensitivity reactions ranging from mild urticaria to life-threatening anaphylaxis. Any type of latex allergy may progress rapidly and unpredictably to anaphylaxis. The reactions are divided into three types: local irritation, immediate hypersensitivity, and delayed hypersensitivity.

Local irritation is nonallergic sensitivity that causes dry, crusty skin and is usually resolved with the removal of latex exposure. Delayed hypersensitivity, a cell-mediated or type IV allergic reaction, may manifest within hours to days after exposure and is similar to other types of contact dermatitis (24). The skin may become red, cracked, and blistered; or it can weep fluid, as is found in the rash of poison ivy or nickel dermatitis. The main culprits are the chemicals added during latex processing, which include mercaptobenzothiazole and tetraethylthiuram (also found in nonlatex gloves). Thus, these added chemical ingredients are potentially capable of inducing a delayed-type reaction in users of latex-free products.

The immediate hypersensitivity is an IgE-mediated or type I allergic reaction. It can occur within minutes and is systemic. Clinical signs and symptoms may be itchy eyes, an erythematous papular rash, pruritus, swelling of the lips or tongue, a sensation of impending doom, dyspnea, dizziness, palpitations, diaphoresis, abdominal pain, nausea, rhinitis, asthma, hypotension, and syncope and can ultimately progress to shock and death. The agents responsible for the immediate-type reaction are thought to be naturally occurring proteins in latex. During latex processing, some protein allergens are removed; but the remaining ones adhere to the powder particles, which then act as a vector for aerosol exposure.

Diagnosis

Diagnosis is made initially by the history. Latex-specific IgE testing and skin prick testing may confirm the diagnosis (25). As was mentioned above, a history of atopy, plant allergy, or frequent occupational or surgical exposure may suggest the diagnosis. The differential diagnoses include drug reactions caused by penicillins or contrast dyes and angioedema caused by ACE inhibitors.

Differential Diagnosis

This can include the following conditions:

- Anaphylaxis from any other cause.
- Drug reactions.
- Asthma—occurs without latex exposure.
- Other allergic reactions.
- Other type of contact dermatitis—often with a history of exposure.
- Eczema—lifelong, more common in childhood than latex allergy.
- Psoriasis—affected skin tends to be more white and scaly.

Referral

Referral to an allergist may be necessary to confirm the diagnosis of latex allergy and to exclude other potentially life-threatening allergies. The allergist may choose to pursue possible desensitization to the latex. The primary care physician must also educate the patient or refer the patient for education regarding avoidance of latex and on how to initiate treatment upon exposure.

Management

Management of an anaphylactic reaction to latex is the same as that for any other anaphylactic reaction (see page 165). Protecting the airway is critical. Activation of emergency medical services is appropriate for moderate to severe reactions. Use latex-free materials during the intervention!

Medications

The following interventions should be used for treatment:

- Oxygen. Given via nasal cannula or facemask as needed to maintain oxygenation.
- Epinephrine. Administered subcutaneously, intravenously, or by nebulization. Dose is 0.005–0.01 mg/kg, depending on severity (see page 167).
- Antihistamines. Diphenhydramine, 0.5–2 mg/kg orally, intramuscularly, or intravenously to prevent subsequent progression. H_2 blockers, such as cimetidine, may be substituted if sedation is undesirable, although this represents an off-label use of this drug.
- Steroids. May be given orally, intramuscularly, or intravenously to stop the inflammatory cascade and to prevent progression. Doses in common uses are methylprednisolone, 0.25–2 mg/kg intravenously every 6 hours during the acute phase, followed by prednisone 1–2 mg/kg orally upon arising for several days to reduce the likelihood of a late-phase reaction.

Follow-up

Monitoring the disease course during an anaphylactic reaction implies monitoring vital signs and providing appropriate support. Initial stabilization should be instituted by whomever is available and with whatever materials are at hand while emergency medical services are activated. For less severe reactions, the patient should follow up with the family physician within 24 hours. Potential problems and complications include subsequent and more severe allergic reactions.

Patient Education

Avoidance of latex material is the best prevention strategy (26). Information about latex allergy should be provided to the individual. Only latex-free materials should be used during subsequent examinations and phlebotomy. Physicians caring for latex-sensitive persons must act as their advocates in building awareness of the problem and in developing protocols for their safe care. Latex-sensitive individuals should consider wearing a Medic-Alert bracelet or necklace and should be educated about the latex content of common objects (25).

SUGGESTED READINGS

1. Guha N. Common respiratory emergencies. *J Ind Med Assoc* 1973;61(6): 286-292.

2. Rees H. Respiratory emergencies. *Practitioner* 1973;211(261):17-24.

3. Runge JW, Schafermeyer RW. Respiratory emergencies. *Prim Care* 1986; 13(1):177-192.

REFERENCES

1. Shafer DM. Respiratory emergencies in the dental office. *Dent Clin N Am* 1995;39(3):5410-554

2. Greenberger PA. Contrast media reactions. *J Allergy Clin Immunol* 1984; 74:600.

3. Lieberman P, Siegle RA, Taylor WW Jr. Anaphylactoid reactions to iodinated contrast material. *J Allergy Clin Immunol* 1978;62:174.

4. Mace S, Vadas P, Pruzanski W. Anaphylactic shock induced by intra articular injection of methyl prednisolone acetate. *J Rheumatol* 1997;24(6): 1191-1194

5. Rohrer CL, Pichler WJ, Helbling A. Anaphylaxis: clinical aspects, etiology and course in 118 patients. *Schweiz Med Wochenschr* 1998;128(3): 53-63.

6. Nagy I, Lee TH, Kay AB. Neutrophil chemotactic activity in antigen-induced late asthmatic reactions. *N Engl J Med* 1982;306:497.

7. Reiss M. [Anaphylactic shock. Diagnosis—therapy—emergency measures]. [In German] *Fortschr Med* 1998;116(5):24-30.

8. Schwartz LB, Metcalfe DD, Miller JS, et al. Tryptase levels as an indicator of mast cell activation in systemic anaphylaxis and mastocytosis. *N Engl J Med* 1987;316:1622-1626.

9. Vleeming W, van Amsterdam JG, Stricker BH, de Wildt DJ. ACE inhibitor-induced angioedema. Incidence, prevention and management. *Drug Saf* 1998;18(3):171-188.

10. Rosen P, Barkin RM, eds. *Emergency medicine*, 4th ed. St Louis: Mosby-Year Book, 1992:2761.

11. Planells Roig M, Enguidanos MJ, Vinuesa Vilella MC, et al. [Hereditary angioneurotic edema with exclusive abdominal manifestation. Report of a case]. [In Spanish] *Rev Esp Enferm Dig* 1997;89(8):640-643.

12. Borum ML, Howard DE. Hereditary angioedema. Complex symptoms can make diagnosis difficult. *Postgrad Med* 1998:103(4):251, 255–256.

13. Frank MM, Gelfand JA, Atkinson JP. Hereditary angioedema; the clinical syndrome and its management. *Ann Intern Med* 1976;84:580.

14. Frye CB, Pettigrew TJ. Angioedema and photosensitive rash induced by valsartan. *Pharmacotherapy* 1998:18(4):866–868.

15. Bey D, Browne B. Clinical management of latex allergy. *Nutr Clin Pract* 1997;12(2):68–71.

16. Kelly JK, Walsh-Kelly CM. Latex allergy: a patient and health care system emergency. *Ann Emerg Med* 1998;32:6.

17. Woods JA, Lambert S, Plattts-Mills TA, et al. Natural rubber latex allergy: spectrum, diagnostic approach, and therapy. *J Emerg Med* 1997;15 (1):71–85.

18. Kelly KJ, Kurup V, Zacharisen M, et al. Skin and serological testing in the diagnosis of latex allergy. *J Allerg Clin Immun* 1993;91:1140–1145.

19. Thompson G. Managing latex allergy in hospital patients and health-care workers. *J Wound Care* 1996;5(S-10):1–7.

20. Jensen VB, Rasmussen KB, Jorgensen IM, et al. Latex allergy in children. *Ugeskr Laeger* 1997;159(21):3172–3174.

21. Ho A, Chan H, Tse KS, et al. Occupational asthma due to latex in health-care workers. *Thorax* 1996;51(12):1280–1282.

22. Lundberg M, Wrangsjo K, Johansson SG. Latex allergy from glove powder–an unintended risk with the switch from talc to cornstarch? *Allergy* 1997;52(12):1222–1228.

23. Haynes BF, Fauci AS. Cellular and molecular basis of immunity. In: Isselbacher KJ, Braunwald E, Wilson JD, et al., eds. *Harrison's principles of internal medicine,* 13th ed. New York: McGraw-Hill, 1994:1544–1559.

24. Kelso JM. Latex allergy. *Pediatr Ann* 1998;27:11.

25. Reddy S. Latex allergy. *Am Fam Physician* 1998;57(1):93–102.

26. Salim A, Warin AP. Hypersensitivity reactions to latex in patients having topical treatment applied by health professionals wearing latex gloves. *Contemp Dermatol* 1998;39(1):44–45.

APPENDIX 1

Supplies for Office Emergencies

Equipment

- Nebulizer
- Electrocardiograph
- Automatic external defibrillator
- Bag-valve-mask resuscitator (with child and adult masks)
- Oropharyngeal airway (child and adult sizes)
- Cervical collar
- Bulb syringe
- Obstetric pack
- Splints (miscellaneous sizes)
- Portable suction unit with regulator
- Blood pressure cuff (child and adult)
- Suction catheters (6–14F) with wall or portable suction
- IV catheters (14–24G)
- IV tubing
- Cricothyrotomy kit
- Sterile bandages (2×2, 4×4)
- Suture material (2-0 through 6-0 absorbable and nonabsorbable)

Medications

- $D_{50}W$ (25 g)
- Oxygen (bottled) with delivery device
- Epinephrine (1:10,000; 1:1,000)
- Normal saline or Ringer's lactate (2 L)
- Lidocaine (1%)
- Metaproterenol (5%)
- Bicarbonate IV
- Nitroglycerine (sublingual or ointment)
- Aspirin (baby and adult)
- Proparacaine HCl (0.5%)
- Methylprednisolone (IV and tablets)

A PPENDIX 2

Office Information

- Poison Control Center telephone hotline number(s)
- Illustration of cardiopulmonary resuscitation
- Illustration of Heimlich maneuver
- Illustration of airway
- Names, addresses, and telephone numbers of local area hospitals
- Telephone numbers of local emergency departments and emergency services/ambulance
- Transportation (911) with office address including cross-streets and landmarks

APPENDIX 3

General Emergency Medicine Resources

1. Tintinalli JE, Ruiz E, Krome RL, eds. *Emergency medicine. American College of Emergency Physicians*, 4th ed. New York: McGraw-Hill, 1996.
2. Callahan ML, ed. *Current practice of emergency medicine*, 2nd ed. Philadelphia: BC Decker, 1991.
3. *Wound closure manual*. Ethicon Inc., 1994.
4. Grossman JA. *Minor injuries and repairs*. New York: Gower Medical, 1993.
5. Saunders G, Ho S, eds. *Current emergency diagnosis and treatment*, 5th ed. New York: McGraw-Hill, 1997.
6. Kaplan D, ed. Office urgencies. *Patient Care* 1999;33(3):13–206.

Telephone Resources:
American Heart Association:
1-800-AHA-USA1

REFERENCES

1. Buyre MT, Gobetti JP, Plezia R. A basic approach to management of medical emergencies in the dental office: Part 1. *J Mich Dent Assoc* 1998;80 (1):34–43.

2. Buyre MT, Gobetti JP, Plezia R. Medical emergencies in the dental office: Part 2. *J Mich Dent Assoc* 1998:80(2):52, 56–59.

3. Kaplan BR. Treatment of medical emergencies for the general practitioner. *R I Dent J* 1994:27(4):5–7.

4. Lipp M, Kubota Y, Malamed SF, et al. Management of an emergency: to be prepared for the unwanted event. *Anesth Pain Control Dent* 1992;1(2): 90–102.

5. Malamed SF. Back to basics: emergency medicine in dentistry. *J Calif Dent Assoc* 1997;25(4):285–286, 288–294.

6. Schexnayder SM, Schexnayder RE. 911 in your office: preparations to keep emergencies from becoming catastrophes. *Pediatr Ann* 1996:25 (12):664–666, 668, 670, passimtr.

7. Fuchs S, Jaffe DM, Christoffel KK. Pediatric emergencies in office practices: prevalence and office preparedness. *Pediatrics* 1989:83:931–939.

8. Altieri M, Bellet J, Scott H. Preparedness for pediatric emergencies encountered in the practitioners office. *Pediatrics* 1990;85:710-714.

9. Flores G, Weinstock DJ. The preparedness of pediatricians for emergencies in the office. *Arch Pediatr Adolesc Med* 1996;150:249-256.

10. Schweich PJ, DeAngelis C, Duggan AK. Preparedness of practicing pediatricians to manage emergencies. *Pediatrics* 1991;88:223-229.

11. Shetty AK, Hutchinson SW, Mangat R, Peck GQ. Preparedness of practicing pediatricians in Louisiana to manage emergencies. *South Med J* 1998;91(8):745-748.

12. Herranz JB, Hernandez MR, Caceres GR, et al. Pediatric emergencies in a community health center. *An Esp Pediatr* 1997;47(6):591-594.

SUBJECT INDEX

Note: Page numbers followed by an *f* indicate figures; those followed by a *t* indicate tables.